12.78 To Jot

MW00715898

I Can!

Discovering the Real Truth
About Change

Rita —
Love our Sundays
together!
Blessings!
Marily

Other Books From Total Sculpt

8-Week Makeover for Body & Soul

by Marilyn Jeffcoat

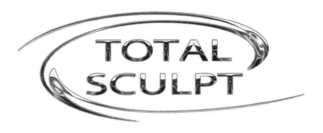

Total Sculpt is a holistic program that incorporates body and soul sculpting exercises to achieve fitness from the inside out.

Founded by Marilyn Jeffcoat, who lost 100 pounds in one year by applying the Total Sculpt principles, the program blends vigorous cardio and weight workout routines with penetrating biblical life-coaching studies to shape every dimension of an individual.

Total Sculpt classes have made dramatic differences in people's lives — weight loss, improved health, and deeper trust in Christ.

**For more information, visit www.totalsculpt.com
or call 1.888. 9 SCULPT**

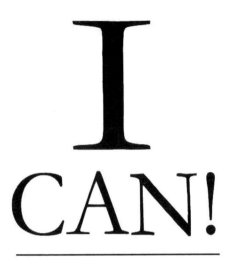

I
CAN!

Discovering the Real Truth
About Change

Marilyn Jeffcoat
Gregory P. Samano, II, D.O.
David Uth, Ph.D.

Punch Press
3143 S. Stratford Road, Winston-Salem, NC 27103-5825
www.punchbookstore.com

© 2005 by Marilyn Jeffcoat, Greg Samano, II, and David Uth. Published by Punch Press.

All rights reserved. No part of this publication may be reproduced in any form without written permission from Punch Press, 3143 South Stratford Road, Winston-Salem, NC 27103.

Unless otherwise identified, all Scripture quotations in the publication are from the English Standard Version (ESV). © Copyright Crossway Bibles, a division of Good News Publishers. Used by permission.

ISBN: 09770807-5-7

Printed in the United States of America

Contents

Part Two: Why "I Can!" Wins

Introduction

The Power of "I Can!"

If the audience I was about to face in a couple of hours had any idea, I would be too ashamed to face them. This was supposed to be a defining day in my ministry. I should have been on top of the world. Many had invested so much of themselves to help me launch this new conference ministry. Finally, the day had come for this inaugural conference session.

I awoke early so that I could run through my talk, which was geared to motivate and inspire others to action. I made sure I had my illustrations nailed. Also, I had interspersed humor to help offset the intensity of the message—and to keep me enough removed from the content so that I could maintain an "I'm-a-mature-leader-who-has-her-act-together" façade. No problem. I had worked on this content a long time. Surely I could pull this off and appear as if speaking to large crowds was effortless for me.

But when I laid aside my manuscript to sit quietly before God for a few moments, the tears flowed. God could see through it all: I wasn't the person that I was planning to project to those women. He forced me to stop and take such a long look at myself that, even now, as I type these words, every detail of those moments returns with such clarity of memory—and grips my heart with such intensity—that I choke to fight back the tears.

My Story

I felt like such a phony as I tried so hard to keep the real me hidden. Oh, I could easily admit that I am a miserable sinner who is as screwed up—if not more so—than the next person. I've given up on trying to pretend to be anything else. But what I tried to keep hidden was the deep hurting inside of me. It was too embarrassing to admit that I didn't have it all together. My heart's desire was—and is—to encourage others in the faith. However, at that point in time, there wasn't enough encouragement on the planet to make me feel good about myself. Because I had acted out habitually to anesthetize the pain of having so many life dreams dismissed by others or dashed by disappointment, I hated the person I had become. Joy and excitement were not the emotions filling my heart as I prepared for my big day. Instead, I felt awful inside.

Soon I would face hundreds of women to share with them a message of hope and encouragement. If they only knew how utterly defeated I felt at that moment. When I looked in the mirror, I was ashamed of my obesity and prematurely aged appearance. Every joint in my body ached, and it had become harder and harder to keep going in my physically unfit condition. I felt whipped and powerless to change.

Being "the professional" that I was, I pulled it together, and got ready to go. I squeezed my heavy legs into thick, black tights (size: 3X), put on my monochromatic outfit of ankle-length black skirt and black turtleneck, and then put on a brightly-colored blazer (which I had to duct-tape underneath to keep the front from flying open while I spoke). I did my best to hide the fat—and my pain.

Once in front of the group, I turned it on. I went straight into perky Marilyn mode. God was good and anointed our time together. Many later expressed how God was working on their heart during our time together—especially one lady: my prayer intercessor for the conference, Ruthie Attaway.

Afterwards I was signing some books and speaking to the ladies, when Ruthie approached. I said something to her—something unusual, other than "Hi, Ruthie"—and she responded in an unanticipated way: "Marilyn, while I was in the back of the room praying for you, God laid something on my heart that he wanted me to share something with you. I told him that I did not want to share this with you. But the Holy Spirit kept prompting me to do so. So, I told God that if he truly did want me to share this with you that he would have you greet me in a specific, unusual way." [Note: I cannot remember exactly what the unusual greeting was that she prayed for, but apparently I said it as she approached me. All I remember is the look of shock and then panic on her face.]

"Well, Honey," Ruthie continued to explain, "That is exactly what you said to me when I walked up! So, now I have to share with you what God told me to tell you. Now, understand that I think I am the last person who should be telling you to do this. However, God told me to tell you this—and I have been struggling with him back there the whole time you were speaking. Honey, you are supposed to give up sugar. In fact, you are supposed to give up all white starches. That is going to take the weight off of you."

If someone other than Ruthie had said that to me at any other time, I would have been offended—and probably defensive. I never discussed my weight with anyone. Ruthie had no idea the private battle I had been fighting just a few hours earlier. Nor did she know that I had been praying every day that God would help me change and get my eating under control. Because I knew this incredible woman of God truly had been interceding in prayer for me, I received with an open heart what she said as a word from God to me.

The next day I gave up sugar and other white starches—completely. As I believed God was absolutely involved in my doing this, I had a greater motivation and desire to follow through. I was determined to do it. God honored my decision, and empowered me to stick with it. I did not cheat—or even want to cheat—until I reached my goal weight and I had my eating under control. Quickly the weight began to melt away. I immediately began to feel better about myself—as well as feel like change might be truly be possible this time.

I Can! with a Negative Twist

Over the next few weeks and months, my life verse, Philippians 4:13—*I can do all things through Christ who strengthens me*—took on new meaning for me as I began to better understand and apply this truth to my life. "I can do all things" is a powerful concept. When understood in the context of the letter written by Paul to the Philippians, this promise from God can radically change a person's thinking in positive ways. However, taken out of context, and adopted as some kind of self-help motto, it has the potential to promote an unhealthy belief system that can contribute to self-destructive behavior. The latter was my history with this verse.

In high school and college I had adopted this verse as my mantra, which reflected the overarching philosophy of life. There were a number of problems with this—with one of the most obvious flaws being in the way I unpacked the verse. At some point over those years, I shifted the emphasis from "do all things through Christ" to "I can do all things." Rather than seeking to operate under Christ's strength in all things, I began to rely on my own power and abilities.

All my life I had been told, "Marilyn, you can be anything or do anything you want in life." And I bought into it—especially when that message was reinforced by the emergence of the "liberated woman" philosophy of the seventies. I became the "I am woman, hear me roar" female. And while I am still a champion of equality for women, I have had to reexamine the application of that message in my life in light of God's Word.

I still agree with the idea that I am capable of doing anything that is my passion. However, that became problematic when I no longer relied on the help of God or waited on his timing in my life. Instead, self-sufficient, Supewoman-me would regularly move forward with my agenda under my own strength to make something happen.

I am sure you can guess what happened—especially to me as a woman in ministry in the Southern Baptist denomination. Doors did not swing wide open for me to pursue a traditional career path in church ministry. One life dream after another was shattered—and the hurt and disappointment got harder and harder to handle. I got good at figuring out alternative ways to do ministry. However, too often, I was impatient and would not wait on God to do what he wanted to do in and through my life. And that would lead to self-destructive patterns of behavior.

I Can! with Positive Results

This time was different. The body change was accompanied by a change of heart. Incredible healing—a healing of the past—took place in my life. The hurt and discouragement from the disappointments and failures in my life began to fade. Anger and bitterness—which I never could acknowledge until the healing process was well underway—radically diminished and was supernaturally replaced with a greater portion of the fruit of God's Spirit: peace, patience, love, joy, goodness, faithfulness, gentleness—and self-control (Gal. 5:22-23). More and more of Christ in me was being outwardly manifested in my life. I was truly being transformed from the inside out!

With every pound I lost, I seemed to lose a pound of life baggage, if you know what I mean. As I cared for the physical me—first through healthy eating, soon followed by regular exercise regime, and then by other means of taking care of myself—I began to like "me" more. The more I liked myself, the more I let people see the real me.

A treasured friend, Dwight Bain—who is a Christian counselor and life-coach—made this observation after seeing me and visiting with me for the first time after I had taken off a big chunk of weight: "Marilyn, I love you with the bubble-wrap off." He went on to explain how he thought the physical change was a nice accomplishment, but he had a greater appreciation for the change that had occurred on the inside of me… as the bubble-wrap was removed from around the me inside.

Over the months and years since these physical and non-physical changes have taken place in my life, I have once again adopted Philippians 4:13 as my life verse. However, this time, I am applying the entire verse to my life. I truly believe I can do all things, but now I have learned the hard way that I can only do those things through Christ. The emphasis is now on Christ and not on Marilyn. I am filled with hope and optimism because of what God is doing in my life.

What's Your Story?

So often when we are told that we can change, we don't really buy into it. Instead, of believing "I can!," all we accept as the truth is our own negative self-talk:

5

Change? Yeah, sure.
I've tried and failed so many times. I've about given up.
I can? I don't really believe it anymore.
You don't know me. No matter...
> *how badly I feel about the person I've become,*
> *how much I really want to change,*
> *how many times I've tried in the past*
...I haven't been able to do it.
I am so weak. I quickly give in to temptation.
I lack willpower. Change never lasts.
I just can't do it on my own.

What Part One of This Book Can Do for You

More than a year ago, I began discussing the idea of collaborating on a book with Total Sculpt medical consultant, Greg Samano, II, D.O. What I envisioned was our writing a book that physicians like him could put into the hands of patients who struggled with positive life change—especially in the area of healthy eating and exercise habits, and that Total Sculpt could offer to individuals and groups for study.

Dr. Samano first developed the Healthy Eating Plan (Appendix B), which he uses with his patients and that we have been testing—with outstanding results—with our Total Sculpt participants. I then asked him to come up with the eight "I Can't" claims—pertaining to making healthy eating choices—that he hears most often from patients. These are the half-truths that many of us tell when we are side-stepping the real issue of why we can't realize the change we desire. In fact, some of these statements may be exactly what you have said to your physician. Dr. Samano really nailed these!

We took these things that you and I say, and began each of the eight chapters in Part One with one of these claims. Then Dr. Samano and I answered each of those claims with a life strategy to help individuals achieve positive results and lasting change. We then tested this material with our Total Sculpt classes and conferences—and got encouraging feedback. Appropriately applied, these strategies work. They can change your outlook—and your life.

When we had completed this part of the book, we added an exercise tip to round out the chapters for tried-and-true ideas for realizing body success.

Consult your physician. If he so recommends, give the eating and exercise plans a try. Stick to the plans for eight weeks. Take your measurements (Appendix C) before starting and at the conclusion of the 8 weeks. Keep a food and exercise journal (Appendix C).Yes, you can do it!

What Part Two of This Book Can Do for You

My plan from this book's inception was to base the positive message of the book on Philippians 4:13 ("I can do all things through Christ who strengthens me"). After Dr. Samano and I had developed the material for Part One of the book, I began searching the book of Philippians for eight "I Can!" biblical truths that could be applied to each of the chapters in Part One.

I rejoiced when God quickly led me to two scriptural passages in each of Philippians' four chapters that perfectly matched up with the eight claims and strategies. I then wrote eight brief lessons from Philippians, which we also used in our Total Sculpt classes.

When it came time to expand the content of the Philippians lessons into book chapters, I asked Dr. David Uth (with a Ph.D. in New Testament) to collaborate with me on this part of the book. Dr. Uth has a fabulous command of Scripture, as well as Greek (the language of the New Testament). In addition to that, he's "normal"(not a stuffy pastor or academician)—and can apply the truths of God's Word in a way that we all can relate. Pastor David was a great writing "fit" for our team. I love what God produced in these chapters: encouraging, uplifting truth based on his Word.

The eight chapters in Part Two correspond to the same chapter in Part One. You can choose to read and study both parts of the book simultaneously, sequentially, or independently. If you are just looking for a Bible study for personal or group use, skip Part One and go straight to Part Two. The eight chapters (of both parts) also work well as a weekly study.

You Can Change

You can change. It is never too late. Your past track record doesn't matter. And even better, you are not alone or left to your own resources. God understands your human condition, your constant struggle with temptation, and your limited ability to change. And he has made provision for these.

The book of Philippians offers a message of hope for all who want to move beyond their present condition and become the person they desire. Although written by the Apostle Paul from a jail in Rome (A.D. 62), this letter to the first church in Europe provides encouragement and direction for individuals who struggle with making positive, lasting change in their lives.

I, along with my co-authors, Greg and David, have been praying for you long before your eyes ever read these words. It is our prayer that you will filter every claim, strategy, and tip through the truth of God's Word before applying any of "I Can!" to your life. Pray about it. Ask God to create a "new you"—inside and out. And then get started! Blessings!

–Marilyn Jeffcoat

Part One

"I Can't"

versus

"I Can!"

Introduction

"I Can't" versus *"I Can!"*

Living a healthy lifestyle is sometimes challenging, but by no means impossible. It is certainly an attainable goal—and absolutely worth the effort. The greatest difficulty arises when making the transition from one's current lifestyle to a healthier one. People often set the long-term goal of being healthy without having a long-term mindset. They want quick fixes and fast solutions. Everyone wants huge results minus the huge effort. However, transitioning to a healthier lifestyle isn't always about colossal life change. We often intimidate ourselves when drawing up our life plans by assuming immediate and complete transformation.

As a physician, I believe the small choices we make everyday have a powerful effect on our health and wellbeing. Our everyday decisions—the little habits we don't even realize—make up the lifestyle that we are currently living. Tiny changes such as cutting out soda, eliminating the "white menace" (white bread, white rice...), or playing sports rather than watching them, can have a greater effect than people realize. Remember that weight loss and improved fitness occur as the result of making small, intentional, daily decisions.

Many people will continue looking for an "easy answer" or a "magic bullet" to solve their problems. This is apparent from the vast array of weight loss pills, medicines, and secrets that are constantly marketed to consumers. But long-lasting change will not be realized through these "solutions." In my opinion, the answer is simple but not necessarily easy. A low-starch diet combined with a sustainable exercise regimen will result in dramatic health benefits over time.

But living a healthy lifestyle isn't just about eating right or exercising occasionally. It is way of thinking, of caring for yourself, inside and out. One of the biggest obstacles people have to overcome when attempting life change is themselves. We have a tendency to beat ourselves up, to be negative thinkers. Patients are always coming in complaining about everything that they cannot do. They are so discouraged that they do not even allow for hope. But nothing good can come of constant negative thinking.

Negative thinking will result in negative results. Without an "I Can" attitude, failure is the only option we offer ourselves. This book offers a positive spin on some of the things people tend to think they simply cannot do. For every "I Can't" there is an "I Can." Do not believe the lies that society and negative people in your life tell you. You can do all things through Christ. You just have to decide if you are going to allow Christ to do all things through you.

I hope this book will be an encouragement to you as you change the areas in your life that could work better for you. Positive thinking is one of the biggest keys to successful change in a person's life. You can be healthier. You can improve yourself. You can change bad habits to good. Your job is to be obedient in terms of caring for yourself. Your job is to take action. Begin by eating a little less and moving a little more each day. If you stick with this plan, you will be pleased with the long-term results. So take action, and leave the results to God.

–Greg Samano, II

I
CAN!

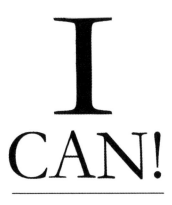

I Can't Claim #1:
I can't seem to lose weight no matter what I do.

Often patients say to me, "I can't seem to lose weight no matter what I do." The explanation that follows is usually along the lines of *I don't know why I have all this weight staying on me. I don't eat that much.* Then, when I ask them to give me an idea of what they normally eat or I look over their food journal, it becomes evident fairly quickly why they are losing the battle of the bulge. They are living in denial of what is the truth about their eating habits. The truth is they are...

*   not thinking carefully about what is going into their mouth.
*   consuming more than they imagined.
*   eating calorie-dense foods with little nutritional value.
*   not sticking with a single healthy eating plan.
*   "cheating" too often.

Many individuals will start with a diet plan and then get frustrated because they are not achieving the results that they want in the time they expected. And they throw the proverbial baby out with the bath water. They give up on the eating plan and begin eating indiscriminately. This often triggers a very destructive cycle of eating excessively followed by extreme dieting and on and on.

It is important to find a single healthy eating plan that is compatible with your needs and lifestyle—and then stick to it. Too often I see people take advice on dieting from varying sources and try to mesh these plans into one nutritional scheme or diet. Frequently these components are low fat, low carb, and low calorie. This creates an impossible diet plan that can never be followed for any length of time. While well-researched studies have shown that each of these three plans work well to varying degrees, they are, however, all mutually exclusive. The three approaches should not be rolled up into one diet.

When looking for a explanation for a lack of weight loss, I find that many patients are eating diets very high in starch. This produces large amounts of insulin in the body. Insulin is responsible for fat production and fat storage. In fact, a roll before dinner will cause most of the meal to be stored as fat.

Also, many people have one or two areas in which they "cheat." Done on a daily or fairly regular basis this can short-circuit even the best weight-loss plan. Examples of this include soda, ice cream, and fast food. Let me add to this line of thinking that I have yet to see someone successfully lose weight drinking diet soda. As yet, I do not have an explanation or mechanism for this. But I just have not seen anyone be successful drinking diet soda.

I Can! Strategy #1:

I can admit that my choices have gotten me where I am.

The first *I Can!* strategy is to admit that your choices have brought you where you are today. Your habits have significantly contributed to the shape you are in.
Your eating choices…
    Your exercises practices…
        Your health maintenance routines…
            Your rest and sleep habits…
                Your sexual lifestyle…
                    Your substance decisions…

All of these choices—and count-
less many more—have shaped you
into the person you have become.
Fess up. Abandon thinking:
* *I'm a victim.*
* *I'm not responsible for where I
  am today.*
* *I don't have what it takes to
  change.*
* *I'll always be this way.*

Admit that you are responsible for the choices you make:
* You alone are responsible for
  what goes in your mouth.
* You alone are responsible for
  what you do to get in shape.

Did you know?

A recent study found
that, all else being
equal, people who
drank one regular soda
a day gained over
twenty pounds in eight
years compared to
non-soda drinkers.

*Journal of the American
Medical Association*
(Aug. 25, 2004), 292(8): 927-934.

* You alone are responsible for meeting your health needs.
* You alone are responsible for getting adequate rest.
* You alone are responsible for your sexual practices.
* You alone are responsible for saying "no" to substances.

Your choices have brought you where you are today. If
you are getting poor life results, look the choices you have made
that have yielded this outcome. Are you where you want to be?
Are you where you want to stay?

Realize that if you do not change the way you think and
the choices you make, you will continue to get the same results.
Take action. Assume responsibility for your choices. Change begins on the inside... with your thinking... with your choices.

Put it into practice.

Keep a food journal and share it with someone to
whom you will be accountable. Without changing
your eating habits, keep an eating log so that you
might accurately evaluate where you stand.

I Can't Exercise Tip #1:

I can't seem to lose weight no matter what I eat.

Nobody likes to diet. Anyone who is honest will tell you that getting started is difficult, and remaining faithful to a diet is tough. Everyone has cravings, everyone has weaknesses. However, the resulting benefits often outweigh whatever sacrifices have been made.

But sometimes, simply eating right isn't enough. Sometimes sacrificing our favorite foods doesn't have the dramatic effect we're hoping for when we step back on the scale. This can be a frustrating phenomenon, but one that can be dealt with. The key to losing weight and living a healthy lifestyle doesn't depend solely on what you put in your mouth. It also has a lot to do with how active you are.

Exercise is imperative. You can't expect to achieve all of your body goals only by changing the way that you eat. You've got to DO something. Regular exercise is a fundamental part of living a healthy lifestyle. If you want to see physical change, if you want the weight to come off, exercise is the missing link.

If regular exercise is not a natural addition to your already busy life, accountability is important. Group exercise classes are a great way to forge new friendships and usually include built-in accountability. If you sign up for an 8-week class, people are going to wonder where you are if you don't show up. But remember, while an exercise program is a great way to start, an active lifestyle doesn't end there.

- Find a sport to play instead of watching sports on TV.
- Visit with friends while walking around the block instead of hanging out on the couch.
- Swim laps instead of lying by the pool.
- Walk during your lunch break instead of sitting around.

Look for ways to be active! Incorporate regular exercise into your week. You will feel better, and be healthier. Combining exercise with healthy eating is a surefire way to lose weight and move towards living a healthier lifestyle.

I CAN!

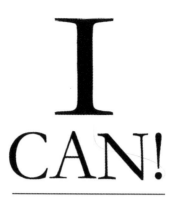

I Can't Claim #2:

I can't stay on a diet.

Patients who struggle with altering their eating habits often have many reasons why they cannot accomplish their goals. Some of their claims usually include:

- *I can't stay on a diet.*
- *I can't stick to a healthy eating plan and feed my family.*
- *I can't control what I eat when I am out with friends.*
- *I can't change the way I eat forever.*

Yes, it is hard to imagine permanently changing a habit—especially one like eating, which we must continue to do multiple times a day and which is the center of so much of our social activity. Forever? Most of us don't have that kind of willpower.

So many of us enthusiastically try a new diet and then give up after only a short time, whenever temptation to cheat or boredom with their plan overtakes our determination to eat healthily or lose weight.

Sheer willpower is not enough. While it does require strong resolve for us to determine we "are going to do it this time," our lack of stick-to-it-ness requires more than mental toughness to stay on a diet.

Diets do not work. Statistics bear out this truth:

- At any given time, 29% of men and 44% of women are on a diet.
- Yet 64% of the U.S. population is overweight or obese.
- Eight out of ten over 25's are overweight.
- Obesity kills more people than drugs, alcohol, guns, AIDS, pollution, and car accidents combined.
- Obesity now rivals tobacco as the top preventable killer in the United States.
- 70% of cardiovascular disease is related to obesity. (According to the American Heart Association, five times more women die of cardiovascular disease than breast cancer.)
- 80% of Type II diabetes is related to obesity. (There has been a 76% increase in Type II diabetes in adults 30-40 years old since 1990.)
- 26% of obese people have high blood pressure.

The American fad dieting approach is failing miserably. Simply putting certain foods in one's mouth at prescribed times of the day will not correct what needs to be "fixed" in that person to insure success in changing their eating habits and the physical fitness of their bodies.

A better plan—a plan that works—is desperately needed by our nation, which is experiencing a rapidly escalating diet-induced health crisis.

I Can! Strategy #2:
Just for today, I can do this.

Chocolate or yogurt? Cookies or fruit? Chips or almonds? French fries or broccoli? Pizza or grilled chicken? One thing is certain: Whether we are "dieting" or not, we will constantly be faced with choices about what to eat. There is no such thing as a one-time decision to change our unhealthy ways. Rather, it is a continuous series of choice after choice after choice.

For diets to work, we need to toss the ideas that a particular diet offers a magic panacea. Instead, we need to find a healthy eating plan that meets our particular physical needs, suits our personality and lifestyle, and offers enough delicious varieties of food that we can stick with it for the long run. Then we need to set manageable short-term goals that help us attain our long-term goals.

A wise, well proven, short-term goal for changing your eating habits would be striving to change your eating behavior one day at a time. While the process is life-long, it only has to be tackled one day at a time, one meal at a time, one food choice at a time. Embrace the thought: *Just for today, I can eat this way.* Then make a no-fail meal and snack plan for that day—and stick to it.

Did you know?
_____

The average American consumes 158 pounds of sugar and 63 pounds of fat per year.

USDA data as cited in "Sugar Intake at an All-time High in 1999," CSPI Newsroom (May 18, 2000).

It has taken years to get your body in the condition it is today. The process of reversing poor eating (and exercise) habits may take some time. When making these new, daily behavioral choices, your body may respond differently than it has in the past. The physical change may be almost overnight and quite dramatic. Or it might be slower, less dramatic process for you—taking you months or even years to realize your long-term goals. Remember: This process is life-long. However, you only have to tackle it one 24-hour segment at a time.

Simple changes made on a daily basis will produce exponential results when performed over the course of your lifetime. No matter what your long-term fitness goals are, eating healthily and exercising regularly will reduce stress, help prevent a variety of life-altering or -ending diseases, give you more energy, and add, on average, about ten years to your life expectancy. Go ahead. Begin with the next choice. Just for today, you can do it!

Put it into practice.
_____

Make your home and work environments as safe as possible. Remove poor food choices and replace with delicious, healthy options.

I Can't Exercise Tip #2:

I can't stick with an exercise program.

Exercise is hard work. It can be grueling. It requires energy and sweat. But the results are tangible. A difference can be made if you are committed to making the effort. Unfortunately, a willing spirit isn't always enough to keep us involved. Sticking with an exercise program is no easy task. So don't be fooled into thinking that there is something wrong with you if you are struggling to commit.

Whenever exercise programs are advertised on TV, they look easy and ensure quick results: 8 minutes to this, 5 minutes to that... In reality, results require hard work and commitment. There is no quick fix when joining an exercise program that will guarantee an easy road to a new you. So beware of those programs promising a pain-free solution. Likewise, there is no shortcut to living a healthy lifestyle. However, as you have hopefully realized, attaining and maintaining a healthy lifestyle, including exercise, is worth the effort required.

So, with that in mind, here are a few ways in which you can overcome the urge to quit, and avoid falling for the latest way to lose weight without even trying.

1. Join a class with a time frame. You will be more likely to participate in something for which you have paid that cannot be made up if missed. No one likes to waste money.

2. Exercise with a friend. Accountability is a huge part of continuing with an exercise program. If you are missed when absent, you will be more likely to attend when possible.

3. Gauge your progress. Don't depend on a scale alone to tell you how you're doing. Taking you measurements before and after exercising over a period of time is far more encouraging. Inches can be lost without fluctuation in weight.

4. Don't give up! Allow time to get used to a program. If you decide early on that you cannot do something, you cheat yourself. You will be surprised after a few weeks of training how exercise becomes more natural and even easier.

I
CAN!

I Can't Claim #3:

I can't stop craving my favorite foods.

When patients struggle with sticking to a healthy eating plan, they often cite needing or craving favorite foods as their major stumbling block. They will share with me the way they think:

- *I have a headache: I need a caffeine fix.*
- *I'm feeling tired: I need some sugar.*
- *It's that time of the month: I need some chocolate.*
- *I'm getting grumpy: I need (real—not diet) food.*

Patients often look to their favorite, unhealthy foods to solve their problems throughout the day. However, this kind of reasoning does not provide the solution to feeling better.

Though your favorite foods may provide you with some form of instant gratification–such as a sugar-, caffeine-, or carbo-hydrate-high–that high will ultimately be followed by a low–and a few extra pounds.

Mind over stomach. Is it possible for your mind to win the battle over the cravings you feel as the day progresses? A mental shift must be made before any physical modifications are even feasible. You must come to the realization that the things you put into your mouth will have an effect on your body. Once that awareness settles in, you begin to assume responsibility for the

21

things that you eat. Think: *Is that food the solution to what I am feeling?*

Managing your cravings is not an easy task. It requires continued commitment as you never know when a craving will rear its ugly head. Remember that cravings don't just go away. However, they can be controlled and even replaced. So, why not just try?

Did you know?

51% of Americans confess to craving comfort foods at least one to three times a day.

According to the national Country Crock Side Dishes Comfort Food Survey.

I Can! Strategy #3:

I can find positive, satisfying habit replacements.

Yes, why not just try? Give it a month or try this plan for eight weeks. It may be easier than you think to replace poor, old habits with positive and satisfying new habits. Here are a few things you might want to try:

- Get in the habit of eating breakfast.
- Don't starve yourself.
- Eat more frequently—and reasonably.
- Delay gratification until mealtime.
- Get rid of any problematic foods.
- Keep delicious replacement foods on hand.
- Don't eat in front of the TV, out of a box, or in the car.
- Stop and think before—and while—you eat.
- Savor each delectable bite.
- Chew gum.
- Drink water, coffee, or tea before a meal.
- Replace late-night snacking with a cup of herbal tea.
- Low-sugar yogurt can be a substitute for ice cream.
- Nuts do a good job in taming a sweet tooth.
- Fresh fruit is a great substitute for breads.
- Spinach works as a replacement for potatoes or pasta.
- Eat more veggies (except corn and potatoes).
- Make healthier carb choices.
- Make healthier protein choices.
- Make healthier fat choices.

Being rested also helps in making food decisions. When you are fatigued, it's hard to make good eating choices. Also, if you get overly hungry, it's hard to stick to an eating plan. If you are starving, you create a state where you will have difficulty in resisting your cravings.

Implement some, if not all, of these ideas into your eating plan. Having a plan for replacing old habits with new habits and sticking to it are the keys to successful eating and weight loss/management. You can do it!

Quote this.

All the resources of the Godhead are at our disposal.

–Jonathan Goforth

Put it into practice.

Studies show that people will eat 25% more, on average, in a single meal when more variety is available. Reducing food selections to three on your plate at a mealtime may prove useful in helping you control your caloric intake.

I Can't Exercise Tip #3:

I can't stop wasting my energy.

Often we cite time as one of the main hindrances to working out regularly. However, lack of energy is usually involved as well. We exert precious energy all day long, and on what? Imagine what in your life simply wears you out. Picture the part of your day when you are being drained of the most energy. Where is your energy going? Is it possible that your energy is not going towards anything at all? That it is simply being wasted on whatever comes your way throughout the day?

- A cranky co-worker
- A rude phone call
- An insensitive family member
- A forever-red traffic signal
- A demanding conversation
- A long line when you are running late
- A misunderstanding

We've all had conversations that make us tired. We've all had moods ruined by a series of red lights. But whatever is draining you of energy unnecessarily needs to be alleviated. While these situations and encounters cannot always be avoided, they can be handled in a healthier, less draining way.

It is a decision that you must make at the start of every day. You can choose to let life happen, and accept what comes your way without pouring yourself into every problem that surfaces. Be as selfish with your energy as you are with your time. Do not waste your energy on things that are of no consequence.

You can and must save your energy so that you can spend it on people and activities that matter to you. In terms of exercise, if you continue to struggle with reserving energy throughout the day, it may be better for you to exercise first thing in the morning. Not only will this guarantee a higher energy level, it will also give you a much-needed boost of adrenaline to start your day.

I
CAN!

I Can't Claim #4:

I can't imagine my life not revolving around food.

Life is series of social gatherings. People are constantly moving from one event to the next, juggling multiple social circles and friend groups. And at the center of most of these events is food. When people gather, people eat. Eating not only provides an excuse for getting together, but also becomes the built-in icebreaker.

Relationships and food go hand in hand. The line *Everyone's got to eat!* has probably helped secure more dating invitations than any other. Consider the cycle of a typical relationship:

1. A relationship begins over coffee.
2. It progresses to drinks or dessert.
3. It continues over popcorn and candy at the movies.
4. It escalates over romantic, candlelit dinners.
5. It solidifies with holiday dinners with the family.
6. It climaxes with wedding cake and a toast.

Life revolving around food is problematic. The problem is not so much in the major events as in the minor events of our lives that have eating at their center. It's the everyday activities dictated and planned according to food that are creating and feeding horrendous eating habits:

- Plans are made over doughnuts in the office break room.
- Friends get together for dinner after work.
- Weekend dinner parties are how connect.
- New neighbors are greeted with baked goods.
- Holidays are based on meals instead of meaning.

It is crucial that you slowly begin to separate your eating habits from your social life. Not all get-togethers require that you eat. And those that do implicitly involve food will simply require a bit of self-control. For example:

- When your friends invite you to go out for ice cream, order the healthiest menu option. (Next time, suggest an alternative gathering place that works better for you.)
- When your family eats out, don't eat everything placed in front of you. (Get in the habit of taking half home.)
- When your co-workers bring doughnuts work, you don't have to finish the box. You can say *No, thanks* and grab a snack.

The key is identifying the times where you are more focused on the food instead of the people with whom you are socializing. Then, determine a way to redirect your attention to healthier options and to interacting with the people in your company. Make people, not food, the center of social events and relationships.

I Can! Strategy #4:

I can set new goals.

If you don't know where you are going,
you will probably end up somewhere else.
–Lawrence J. Peter

When people are dissatisfied with their lives, they have a tendency to stall out. Instead of moving forward, they freeze up or, at best, float along through life. Perhaps, it is because they are convinced that they are stuck and cannot really change anything. That is not a healthy way to think or act.

It is never too late to change. It is never too late to decide where you want to be down the road. It is never too late to move in that direction. Let me suggest three keys to successfully moving forward and realizing change in your life:

26

First, make the decision to change.
Do you really want to change?
- Are you tired of being over-weight?
- Are you tired of feeling run-down?
- Are you tired of living an unhealthy lifestyle?
- Are you tired of making poor life-style choices?

Quote this.

We ought to eat in order to live, not live in order to eat.

–Cicero

Then make the decision once and for all that you are going to do something about it.

Next, come up with a plan for change.
- Nail down your reasons for change. Decide what you hope to achieve through these life changes. Adopt long-term, purposeful living as your mindset and course of action.
- Set new goals for yourself and work hard towards attaining these goals.
- Replace old thinking and habits with new, smart life-choices.

Finally, stick with your plan for change.
Stay with a course of action. For example, when a patient tells me that they are tired of living a life that is food-driven and have made the decision to change, I often suggest they come up with enjoyable alternatives to eating:
- Schedule fun activities into your day and week.
- Be creative pursuing new hobbies. (Sign up for dance class.)
- Pamper yourself with a massage.
- Plan a special outing or trip that revolves around activity.

Adopt these ideas for change into your life. You have the ability to set new goals. You have the ability to dream according to your

Quote this.

If you aim at nothing, you hit it.

–Author Unknown

purpose for change. And you have the ability to act on your desired intentions. The first step is to decide what you want. Then do some-thing about it today. You can lead a happier, healthier life… if you decide that is what you really want.

I Can't Exercise Tip #4:

I can't imagine life not revolving around entertainment.

We belong to a society that expects to be entertained. Whether going to a movie or attending a seminar, our expectations in terms of entertainment are high. Society teaches us to do what feels good. On the contrary, if something cannot keep our attention, if we find ourselves bored, it must not be worthwhile. Unfortunately, our dependence on being entertained has extended into our daily lives and relationships.

Take a good look at your daily life. Once more, evaluate you weekly routine.

- *Do all of your social activities and interactions revolve around entertainment?*
- *Is the majority of your quality time with the people you love spent in front of your television set?*
- *Is a great deal of your time with friends spent in a movie theater?*
- *Are you allowing entertainment to replace truly spending time with people?*
- *Are you allowing entertainment to replace physical activity?*

Letting go of any familiarity can be frightening. You may know the characters of your favorite TV show better than you know members of your own family. It may be difficult for you to imagine an entire day without a show or movie or radio host. But as you are attempting to achieve a healthier lifestyle, there is more involved than eating a little better, and exercising when you can squeeze it in.

Don't cling to excuses formulated by an A.D.D. society. Add depth to your life by eliminating your dependency on being constantly entertained. As a Christian, your life should already be centered around a relationship. Transfer your ability to infuse your relationship with Christ into all aspects of your life. Replace entertainment with people and meaningful activities.

I
CAN!

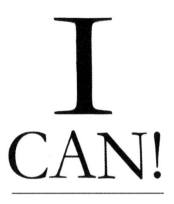

I Can't Claim #5:

I can't find the time for a healthy eating lifestyle.

"I can't find the time." Time is the most common excuse offered by individuals who have fallen into the habit of disregarding their health needs. It is an easy out when confronted with the harsh reality of self-neglect.

- *I can't find time to care for myself.*
- *I can't find time to shop for, much less prepare, healthy meals.*
- *I can't find time to exercise.*
- *I can't find the time to attend to health needs.*

The truth is, it's not the lack of time that is the problem. Rather, it is how we choose to fill the time we have. We all have the same number of hours in our day. While our responsibilities may greatly vary, we control whether or not our commitments rule our lives.

Contemporary culture reveres a lifestyle built around maxed-out schedules. We tend to associate power and importance with how busy someone seems. Too many of us follow suit and allow our schedules to fill up without seriously considering the consequences of constantly being slammed. We lose sight of our priorities and the importance of "me" time.

Instead of claiming you have no time, proclaim that it's the perfect time for you to rearrange your life so that there is time for you to take care of you.

- Abandon the I'm-a-victim-of-my-circumstances mentality.
- Take charge... of your calendar and of your life.
- Juggle, shift, or eliminate appointments as much as possible.

Examine your week day-by-day, hour-by-hour to determine if your time is being monopolized by commitments – big or small – where your presence or participation is not essential. (You may be surprised at how much time you devote to activities that simply do not require your presence.)

As you begin to make the shift to incorporate healthy alternatives and choices into your life, you may find that you have more time than ever on your hands. In fact, most people who exercise consistently experience increased energy, better overall health, and reduced stress. These benefits will multiply your productivity, outweigh the small amount of time invested, and actually put quality time back in your day.

Did you know?

In a survey of 1,200 people by Impulse Research Corporation, 77% of the respondents said that they forego workouts when they get busy.

I Can! Strategy #5:

I can make the time for my true needs.

The hardest part of change is getting started. Start this life shift by saying, "I will make time for my true needs." Then make it a priority to do so. Take comfort in the fact that it is possible for new habits to be established. Also, as these habits are solidified, the benefits will multiply beyond anything you can imagine.
You can become a whole new you...
enjoying a whole new schedule...
providing you a whole new life...
offering whole new possibilities.
You just need to take the time to start living this way!

1. Whole New You. Exercise will yield body results not possible by "dieting" alone. Working out not only burns calories in the process, but also raises your overall metabolism. [Remember: Fat burns very little energy (calories) while muscle burns a substantially greater amount of calories.] Your body was designed to be healthy. It will respond and you can become a whole new you if you commit the time necessary to take care of it.

2. Whole New Schedule. Re-think your life and how you are spending your hours and days. Begin re-shaping each day by eliminating everything that keeps you from functioning at the highest level possible. Within weeks you could be not only operating—but thriving—on a whole new schedule with more time for what really matters.

3. Whole New Life. As you thoughtfully evaluate your life, settle the issue: Are you living the life that God created you to live? Are you intimately connected to God and others in dynamic and growing relationships? Are you handling life's responsibilities and challenges under the control of God's guidance and power or are you letting life control you? Release your burdens, and let God take over and give you a whole new life.

4. Whole New Possibilities. Following the above strategies opens the door to all kinds of new possibilities. Each day should be an adventure. And when your body and soul are strong... and you are living a life under control... you will be up to the task of handling the wonderful opportunities that will come your way.

The key is making the decision to change: to make time for the things that are important... to make time for yourself and your true needs.

Put it into practice.

Studies have shown that people who exercise three times a week live, on average, 10 years longer than those who do not. Get an exercise partner and commit to working out together on a set schedule.

I Can't Exercise Tip #5:

I can't find the time to exercise.

There is never enough time in a day to accomplish everything. Life happens fast, and there will always be something else demanding your attention. You will always be able to come up with an excuse not to exercise if you are looking for it. However, in reality, you have time for everything you make time for in your schedule. In other words, if there is not time in your day for what is most important, you may need to evaluate your day in terms of your priorities.

Whether you realize it or not, your priorities may not currently be reflected by your actions. You spend time on that which you value. Therefore, if you say something is a priority, you should be devoting time to whatever it may be. So if you find yourself running out of time, make an effort to determine where your time had been spent. If you are not spending time on what you care about most, adjustments need to be made. Step one is figuring out where all your time is going.

1. *What do I spend the most time doing every day?*
2. *Whom do I spend the most time with on a daily basis?*
3. *Where do I go most often on an average day?*

If you have trouble answering these question because your day is a blur, perhaps you should try writing down what you do throughout the day. Keeping a "time journal" tracking what you are doing on an hourly basis can be an eye-opening experience for most people. It is surprising how we waste time on insignificant things without realizing that those wasted moments are taking away from something we may enjoy doing.

So the next time you start telling someone that you don't have time to exercise, take a step back. Be honest. There is always time to take take care of your body. Remember, if you do not value yourself enough to be a priority in your own life, you cannot expect to be a priority in somebody else's.

I
CAN!

I Can't Claim #6:
I can't keep from messing up.

"*I was doing fine until...*" " I hear this often as I counsel patients on eating plans and weight loss. They then proceed to explain how they got off to such a great start, began losing weight as they got on track with their new lifestyle choices, felt better than they have felt in a long time, and then they fell victim to . . .

- a major event,
- a social function,
- a family situation,
- a tremendous workload,
- an uncontrollable temptation.

They blame life, others, or some personal shortcoming for their inability to stick with their new way of life. To many, it seems impossible. There's no way they can stick to the plan. Backsliding or failure is inevitable. "I've never been able to do it before . . . " is how the litany begins. And they go on to recount:

All the times they tried to eat healthily . . .
Tried Atkins,
Tried Weight Watchers,
Tried Sugar Busters,
And then they couldn't stick with it.

Did you know?

Findings from a recent study published in the January 5, 2005 *Journal of the American Medical Association* showed that while people can lose weight on popular diet programs, many find it impossible to stick to these eating plans. At the end of one year, 50% had dropped out of the Atkins plan and 35% had abandoned Weight Watchers and the Zone diets. Only 10% of participants had lost and kept off 10% of their initial weight.

All the times they tried to exercise...
    Joined a gym,
    Bought exercise equipment,
    Took up jogging,
And then they quit doing it.

All the times they began seeing results...
    Lost weight,
    Got in shape,
    Felt and look better,
And then they messed up... again.

I Can! Strategy #6:
I can overcome the past.

Have no fear of perfection—you'll never reach it.
–Salvador Dali.

Of course we keep messing up. It's what humans do best. We are imperfect creatures by birth. Our very nature keeps leading us astray. After trying and failing so often, we begin to think:
I can't let go of old habits.
    I can't stop eating my favorite foods.
        I can't make time to exercise.
            I can't change the person I've become.
It is easy to focus on—or even feel defeated by—past failures and the things we have not been successful in changing in our

lives. However, that is not healthy way to think. Yes, we can be certain we will falter again.[1] But this is no reason to be disheartened. Harriet Braiker wisely pointed out that, "Striving for excellence motivates you; striving for perfection is demoralizing."

If we expect perfection from ourselves, then we set ourselves up for failure. We must come to realize that mistakes do not mean our intentions were not good or that we are no good. And past failures do not mean that our present goals cannot be accomplished. They merely are evidence of our humanity.

Mistakes, failures, "messing up" should be expected as you set new goals and move towards them. However, it is important for you to recognize whether this has become a pattern of behavior. If so, do you know why you keep messing up? (Besides your being human.) It is a good idea to consider this before setbacks occur. Then formulate a strategy to cope with the problem.

Finally, when you do mess up, never "throw the baby out with the bath water." Think through what occurred and how to prevent its happening again. Then simply move forward.

Put it into practice.

1. If you're struggling with sticking to your healthy eating plan, you will want to avoid temptation.
2. Then you need to think of and implement a plan.
   - Remove problematic food from your house.
   - Keep fresh fruits and veggies handy for snacks.
   - Don't skip meals allowing hunger to take over.
   - When eating out, don't let the waiter bring breads, chips, or a dessert menu. Replace the temptation with an alternative (a healthy appetizer).
3. Get creative with your food and as time passes your palate will slowly change.
4. If possible, enlist friends or family to help you.

---

[1]Romans 3:10-12.

I Can't Exercise Tip #6:

I can't keep from messing up.

Failure. It will always be a part of our lives. We are imperfect, so mistakes will happen. However, even knowing that failure on some level is inevitable, people allow the fear of failing to incapacitate them. They stop taking risks, they stop trying new things, and they stop living.

It's o.k. to mess up. The question is how we choose to react when it does. Notice that how we react is a choice–it is not involuntary. As you transition from bad to healthier habits, you will struggle. If you're infusing exercise into your schedule for the first time, expect difficult moments.

There will be days when what you want to do does not match up with the lifestyle you want to live. You will want to skip waking up early to go to the gym; to go straight home after work instead of attending an exercise class; to sit on the couch instead of working out. So when those days come, do not beat yourself up. Sometimes those days will get the best of you, and you'll give in to a little lazy pleasure.

The question remains, how will you react to that supposed failure? There are several options, but they can be summer up in three categories.

Option 1: You embrace your mistake. You love and repeat what you know is unhealthy.

Option 2: You feel remorse, but incapable of change. So you allow yourself to continue making mistakes and feeling guilty.

Option 3: You learn from your mistake, move on, and improve yourself based on what you learned.

You must decide ahead of time that messing up, especially in terms of exercising, will not deter you from continuing forward. You must determine that you are committed to achieving a healthier lifestyle, and that you are willing to face and overcome failure from time to time. Life happens. Sometimes the best thing to do is simply get over it!

I
CAN!

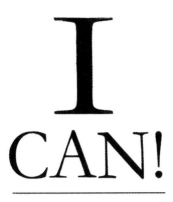

I Can't Claim #7:
I can't seem to get over this plateau.

I have been eating healthily...
I haven't been cheating with sweets...
I initially lost a lot of weight...
But now I have quit losing the pounds.
Why have I stopped making progress?

You did it! You overcame obstacles and made a positive life change. You identified bad habits and swapped them for better choices. You replaced poor food selections with healthy alternatives. You met the challenges in pursuing a new lifestyle and persevered. Pounds and inches were lost. Eating habits were under control. Energy and enthusiasm were high. And now you are stuck!

Welcome to the next phase! This point of your life makeover is often referred to as a plateau. You have been achieving higher and higher levels of results and loving it until... now. You seem to have hit a wall. Everything has come to a halt. And it is so discouraging.

This is common to most who are changing their eating habits and trying to lose weight. Their initial attempts to change will only take them so far. Eventually everyone will reach a point

37

at which their bodies simply get used to their new habits and activities, and quit responding in the same way.

Patients who have been dramatically losing weight and suddenly stopped will come to me and emphatically declare, "I am doing everything right! So why can't I lose any more weight?" I then ask patients a number of questions about their eating habits to determine if some part of their "everything right" is wrong:

1. *How many meals and snacks are you eating each day?*
2. *What are you eating?* (Use a food journal. See Appendix C.)
3. *How much bread do you eat each day?*
4. *How often are you eating pasta? Rice? Potatoes?*
5. *Are you eating any fried foods? Chips?*
6. *How, and how often, do you cheat?*
7. *What times of the day are you eating your meals and snacks?*
8. *How many glasses/cups of water are you drinking each day?*
9. *What else are you drinking, (sodas, lattes, sports drinks)?*
10. *How much fiber are you consuming? In what form?*

It is frustrating to realize that the closer one gets to their ideal body weight, the harder they have to work to ultimately achieve this weight. As hard as it is to get started, it is often harder to finish. Unfortunately, in order to finish, we cannot simply adopt a plan and stick with it. While having a plan is a great place to start, we must always be willing to tweak our plan so that it continues to work for us. We must be willing to change.

I Can! Strategy #7:
I can handle any challenge.

There is no finish line to a healthier lifestyle. It is not a single battle to be won or lost overnight. One of the changes in mindset necessary to maintaining and improving your fitness level is that you are committing to the journey, not a final destination.

So when you reach a plateau, you must simply recognize it as a sign for you to move forward—faster and harder than ever before. As you progress, you will continue to be faced with these challenges, as they are simply part of the process. What is crucial to your success is how you handle the plateaus and other obstacles that are thrown into your path.

Step One. Believe that you can handle any challenge. While some dilemmas are more complicated than others, there is always a solution. There is always a way that you can overcome setbacks and move ahead to achieve significant results.

Step Two. Recognize that your challenges may be unique. You may need solutions that are not simply cookie-cutter answers, but rather are unique-to-you experimentations. It may take some trial and error to see what works best for you. Be patient in finding out what works best for you and your particular needs.

Step Three. Try radical change. In the case of hitting a plateau—one of the most frustrating challenges one will encounter as you make lifestyle changes—the solution is change, radical change. The initial shock your body encountered when you first began to change your eating habits needs to be duplicated. The trick is that in order to shock your body again, you're going to have to try something new. Think of the areas in which you could attempt something dramatic so as to break through the wall you've hit.

Step Four. Don't give up. Take comfort in the fact that everyone must change in order to continue making progress. You have been given the strength to accomplish what you set out to do. All you have to remember is that the road may not always be as smooth as you would like—and that doesn't necessarily mean that you have gotten off-track. And it certainly doesn't mean that you should be discouraged or give up. In fact, you should be excited that you have reached a new level with your body. The need to keep changing is a sure sign that you are making progress. Keep moving forward. Change!

Put it into practice.

Make sure you are truly doing "everything right" and then do it even more "right." Shock your body. For a period of time:

1. Eliminate big meals and try "grazing."
2. Eliminate all bread, dramatically reduce starches.
3. Eliminate all sweets. Don't cheat at all.
4. Drink only water.
5. Substitute a healthy meal replacement drink for a meal.

I Can't Exercise Tip #7:

I can't seem to get over this plateau.

Nothing has changed. I am eating the same things. I am exercising the same amount. Why have the results suddenly stopped?

Sometimes we do everything right, but our results just do not meet our expectations. You may have created a wonderful exercise schedule for yourself. You may be dedicated, not missing a single day of working out. You may even have seen results when you first started. Unfortunately, as we improve our bodies, our bodies become more difficult to improve.

Think of exercising as a form of learning. If you want to learn something when reading a book, you do not just read the first chapter over and over again. Evntually you'll have learned everything there is to learn from that chapter. You will no longer benefit from reading and re-reading it and you will grow bored. That is how our bodies are. When you start exercising, you start at chapter one. Once your body has benefited as much as it can from that chapter, maintenance replaces change. While it's o.k. to remain in chapter one if you are progressing, further improvement requires moving on to chapter two. That transition between chapters often requires "shocking" your body in some way.

This means that in order to continue seeing results you will have to exercise more often and/or more intensely. Your body requires that you take it up a notch if you want to continue making progress. Do not be discouraged. You are not alone. At some point, everyone reaches a plateau.

However, do not expect to reach a plateau at the same point as your friend, spouse, or classmate. Everyone has a unique body, metabolism, and dietary needs. This also means that the way in which you respond to your plateau may be slightly different than those around you. Perhaps your abs are strong, but your arms are weak. You may have to focus on some of your weaker body parts in order to improve yourself overall. The bottom line is you can always do more. You can always be better. But sometimes in order to be better, you have to do more.

I
CAN!

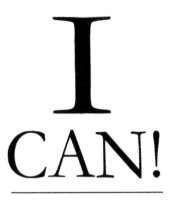

I Can't Claim #8:
I can't believe I can really change.

If you convince yourself
that you cannot change,
Then you are ensuring
that you will not.

The battle to change our self is often lost before change is ever attempted. We thwart plans that have not even been made. We have so little belief in ourselves that we often forgo trying anything at all. We have a chorus of voices in our head telling us all that we cannot do:

I can't overcome my past.

I can't undo whom I've become.

I can't be the person I want to be.

I can't truly change.

Why the negative self-talk? It is much easier to declare something impossible or claim that you will once again fail than it is to embark upon that which probably will be difficult and demand great commitment on your part. If you've convinced yourself that you cannot change, then your worst fears will come true: You won't change… because you won't allow yourself to do so.

Earl Nightingale said, "We tend to live up to our expectations." If we expect failure, then we will live up to that expectation. Yes, we all have to face the failures of our past when considering our future. But that does not mean that we have to be bound by our past.

Of course, you've failed before. Everyone has. The difference is in learning from past failures—and then doing something to correct your life course. It's more than simply de-

> **Quote this.**
> _____
> *It is never too late to become what you might have been.*
> –George Eliot

ciding to be a different person. You need a plan for change—and then stick to that plan. Bad habits don't just go away. They are replaced... with great intentionality and persistence. It also takes tremendous effort as you make better daily choices and sacrifice immediate gratification for long-term benefits.

Take comfort in the fact that believing genuine change is impossible is a common problem. Even more so, be encouraged as the solution is much easier than you may have ever imagined. First, dismiss negative self-talk. Second, focus on that which is true and good: You—with God's help—can truly change your life. Third, risk it! Live as though you have already realized this great change in your life and then make it happen. Become the person you have always wanted to become.

I Can! Strategy #8:
I can expect positive, lasting results.

You can change.
You can improve your life.
You can expect more out of life.
You can be happy with yourself.

Change is only as intimidating at you allow it to be. If you trying to do an overnight 180°, then change is probably a pretty intimidating prospect. However, if you dissect change for what it is—one small choice on top of another small choice—then there's nothing to be afraid of. Positive life change is simply the accumulation of better choices. It occurs one decision at a time, not all at once. You simply need to make a different choice right now . . . and now . . . and now.

Having accepted the idea that change is indeed possible, you can look forward to the ongoing results that will certainly ensue:

- As the months and years pass as you maintain this new life and nutrition plan, your body will become more and more efficient at burning fat and maintaining or losing weight.
- The longer you live out your healthier lifestyle, the more satisfying it will become. Your tastes will change and you will begin to enjoy things you once struggled to embrace (e.g., new food choices, regular exercise).

Yes, you can realize lasting, positive life change.
If this is difficult for you to believe . . .
If it sounds too good to be true . . .
Allow yourself time to be convinced.
Allow yourself the freedom to believe.

Obedience often precedes faith. You absolutely can act your way into right thinking. Stick with your plan. And the results will be there to convince you. If you determine now that you are committed to your new lifestyle, then you truly can expect positive, lasting results.

Put it into practice.

Commit to the new you by:
- Making better choices… one at a time
- Keep practicing new habits.
- Eliminate/flee stumbling blocks.
- Stay vigilant.
- De-stress & rest.
- Try new things.
- Have fun!

I Can't Exercise Tip #8:

I can't believe I can really change.

To change is difficult. Not to change is fatal.
            –Ed Allen

Change doesn't just happen. It requires effort, dedication, and usually a little bit of frustration. When attempting to add exercise to an already full schedule, just the thought can be exhausting. Routines and habits are tough to alter, especially ones that revolve around other people. But change is possible. Plenty of busy people have found ways of incorporating self-care into their daily lives. All you need to do to get started is adopt the mindset that change in your life can and will happen.

There is no guarantee that you won't encounter a few snags as you attempt to reinvent yourself in terms of exercise. In fact, it would be quite unusual if your transition was smooth sailing from start to finish. But you can maintain a positive attitude. One of the most difficult things about trying to change ourselves for the better is the fear of failure. However, we cannot allow negative thoughts to prevent us from trying to improve.

Believing in yourself is one of the most empowering things you can do. If you do not believe that you can change, it is not likely that you will have much support from the people around you. However, if you commit yourself to an exercise program, believe in ability to change, and follow through, you will not be the only one to benefit. Your success will encourage others in ways that you cannot imagine. You will not only be accomplishing your goals, you will be setting an example for other people to do the same.

Believing in yourself is the first step. Continuing to believe in yourself throughout the process is the next. Take on this attitude and you will ensure successful change. Change is possible and exercise can be a part of your every day life.

Part Two

Why
"I Can!"
Wins

Introduction

Why "I Can!" Wins

Life is a trip, isn't it? The life to which I am referring isn't just existing or having a biological life. Instead, it is the life to which Jesus referred when he said, "I am come that they might have life, and that they might have it more abundantly" (John 10:10). For the believer in Jesus Christ the real journey starts the day Christ comes into their life and ends when they are in the presence of the Lord. And the secret to having the abundant life is learning how to enjoy every day in between.

It was never the Lord's intention that the journey not be filled with joy. I have always thought that there's joy in our ultimate destination, because heaven is a great place. It is said that when we die we are going home. Of heaven Paul says, "We eagerly await a Savior from heaven because that is where our citizenship is." Yes, heaven is going to be great. However, don't miss out on all that God's got in store for you for the rest of the trip.

All along the way God has a word for you: He wants you to enjoy the ride. There is so much God is doing right now and even more he wants to do in your life along the way—including the good, the bad, and the stuff that just happens. For some, this is not a problem, but for others life has become so "daily." It takes all of their strength to get up and put one foot in front of the other.

The journey is different for all of us. But there is the one thing we all share in common: We only have a certain amount of days in our journey. And none of us knows how long the journey will be. One day this journey will end.

Imagine a large glass container full of marbles to represent the life of a young child. Imagine that same container with only half of that amount of marbles to represent someone who is middle-aged. Then envision a container holding very few marbles to represent an elderly person.

At best, my container would be the one only half full. As I think about the container that is full of marbles and then imagine mine, I think, "Where did it go?" Even more important, I'm forced to consider: "What am I going to do with the rest of my life?"

A contemporary song writer wrote lyrics following this same line of thinking: "What will you do with the time that's left? Would you live it all with no regret?" I guess I am that mid-life point where I am asking myself these kinds of questions. How am I going to make the rest of my life count for Jesus Christ?

Every one of us has life as a gift. And we are not all guaranteed a container full of marbles. None of us can assume we will have 75 or 80 years before we leave and stand before God. In reality, I don't know that I have all of these marbles left. I would like to think I do! All I know is that my prayer is: "Lord, for every day I have left—for every marble you give me—help me to make it count"

That is exactly why Paul wrote the book of Philippians. He was in a Roman prison and he knew that life was short. Any day they could come and say, "Paul, that's it. Your life is over." Although he had received a word from the Lord that he might be able to go on and have a fruitful ministry, Paul lived with the realization that any day it could be over.

Paul's letter makes me think about this question: What am I going to do with the time that I have left? There is no need for me to talk about yesterday's successes or failures. I would love to go back and put some more marbles in my container. I would love to add back some marbles and say, "Lord, I would like to do my high school years over again. I would like to do college years over. I would like to have some of those months back." But none of us can get them back!

So, all I pray is that for the rest of my life, I will enjoy the journey. I don't want to miss a thing God has for me. If that is your prayer, let's start learning the lessons of Paul from a Roman prison and unlocking the truths about "I Can!"

–David Uth

I
CAN!

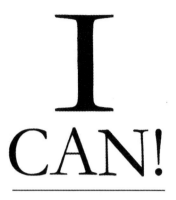

Truth #1:
I can choose to live a life that matters.
Philippians 1:6, 9-11

An evening news report showed heartrending television footage of an airplane crash. As the camera panned the site, there were images of suitcases, shoes, stuffed animals, and other personal property—poignant reminders that these were real people who lost their lives in that fatal crash.

When the jumbo jet hit the ground, the tail section broke off and threw one row of seats from the fuselage. While the main body of the plane turned into a cartwheeling fireball, this row of seats miraculously came to rest in an upright position with its two passengers still strapped in, terrified but relatively unharmed! The televised account told of two survivors unbuckling their seatbelts and walking away from the crash. When interviewed, one of them commented, "This experience has made me stop and reconsider what really matters in my life."[2]

Sometimes it takes a crisis or an illness, the loss of a loved one or the loss of income, a broken heart or a failed marriage to

---

[2] Jim Henry with Marilyn Jeffcoat, *Keeping Life in Perspective* (Nashville: Broadman & Holman, 1996), 1.

cause us to stop and evaluate what is most important to us in life—and whether or not we are pursuing the most important things. Before we get to the point where we are ready to say *"I can,"* we have got to realize and admit *"I need to change."*

So, before you go any further in this study of Philippians, ask yourself:

- *Am I happy with my life?*
- *Am I growing in the important relationships in my life, including my relationship with God?*
- *Am I wasting my time and energy on things that don't really matter, instead of pursuing that which truly matters?*
- *Am I where I want to be at this point in my life journey?*
- *Am I ready to choose to change?*

Life is a process.

We are a work in progress. When we embrace Christ as our Savior and Lord, a "good work" of God is begun in our heart and life:

And I am sure of this, that he who began a good work in you will bring it to completion at the day of Jesus Christ.

—Philippians 1:6

We are made a new creation in Christ (Eph. 2:10). As in creation of mankind, (Gen. 1:31). This new work of God in our life is also "good."

The "good work" of God in our life is not complete at salvation. This transformation process is not made perfect "until the day of Christ Jesus" (Phil. 1:6). And God promises to continue to work in our life until his work in us is completed (v. 6).

God intends that we know the goodness of his work in our life. Joy is not just in the destination of our life journey: the final outcome of and for our life. Joy is to be ours in the journey, in the process of God doing his good work in our life and our seeking what matters most in life.

Life is a gift.

Everyone has life as a gift. While life's journey is different for all of us, we all have this in common: Our days journeying are limited. Life is short, and the time we have on earth is precious. Do we simply mark off the days on our calendar or do we choose to live a life that counts?

You have a choice. What are you going to do with this precious gift? How are you going to live the rest of your life? The choice is yours. You alone are responsible for:

- *your decision about responding to Christ's call to follow him.*
- *your choices about seeking first his Kingdom.*
- *your lifestyle of relating intimately in a love relationship with Christ.*
- *your practice of spiritual exercises to draw you closer to God.*
- *your habits of embracing God's truths for your life.*
- *your routines of Christ-like obedience.*

When you say *I can't make wise, godly choices* are you really saying *I won't*? Saying *I can't* may be some sort of attempt to absolve your self of personal responsibility for your life choices. However, you are responsible. It is up to you to choose to how you will live your life.

Life is choices.

How are you going to respond to life? …and to God and what he can do in your life? You can choose to take God at his Word and live life under his guidance or make decisions based on feelings and the lies of this world.

The Apostle Paul knew that life is short. He was in prison. Any day his life could be over. He urged the readers of this Philippians' letter to pursue what matters most in life, to get passionate about the right things. Paul also prayed a powerful prayer (vv. 9-11) that asks God to help his readers to choose to make their lives count. This prayer of Paul is as much for your life today as it was for his original audience:

And it is my prayer that your love may abound more and more, with knowledge and all discernment, so that you may approve what is excellent, and so be pure and blameless for the day of Christ, filled with the fruit of righteousness that comes through Jesus Christ, to the glory and praise of God.

–Philippians 1:9-11

Paul prays that you should grow in three areas of your life. Each of these three life qualities works together and builds on the others. Paul prays that . . .

1. Your love may abound more and more.

Picture three steps. *"That your love may abound more and more"* (v. 9) is the first or foundational step. It is the foundation of what we are going to ask God to do in us.

The verb used here is in the present tense, which means it is something that should occur continually. No matter how old you are, or how long or how well you have known Jesus, you should always pray that your love abounds more and more. You aren't there yet. You haven't reached the end of what God wants to do in and through your life. You should always pray, "Lord, I want my love to abound more and more."

The phrase "more and more" is used thirty-nine times in the New Testament—with twenty-six of those times its being used by Paul. He loved this phrase. What does it mean to have your love abound more and more? It has to do with passion or pursuit.

However, you have to be careful with the prayer at this point. You need to understand how you should passionately give or pursue love. Paul qualifies this foundational step of his prayer with the phrase: "with knowledge and discernment." Why is your having knowledge and discernment important? Because, there are a lot of things you do not need to be passionate about. It is easy to get carried away. Paul is saying, "Your love and your passions need to be checked by knowledge and discernment, because there are some things not worthy of your love, energy, or passion."

Do you realize that the highjackers who flew the planes into the Twin Towers on 9/11 were very passionate? They were very much abounding in love—love for Allah. It is important to have knowledge and discernment about the way in which we direct our passion and love.

The word Paul uses for knowledge here is *epignosis*, which means an intense technical understanding of something. When Paul combines that term with the word "knowledge," he is saying: "We ought to truly know the object of our love as we continue to get more and more passionate about things that really do matter." Before giving your heart away, ask yourself:

What is the truth about the object of my love?
Is this a wise and godly choice?
Where will this love lead me?
What will be the consequence of my choice?

2. You may approve what is excellent.

This is the phrase in the prayer that really got to me [David]. Paul took a phrase—"what is excellent'—that really belonged to the Stoic philosophers of his day. The Stoics taught that you couldn't change life. As they were very fatalistic, they felt you needed to approach life without emotion. (That is what is meant when we say that someone is stoical.) Whatever came their way, the Stoics just dealt with it.

Paul uses this phrase "what is excellent"—which also may be translated "what matters"—to communicate that we should pray: "Lord, I want to have my love grow in knowledge and discernment so I can approve in my life what really matters. God, help me not to give heart away or passionately pursue things that are not worth it."

I think that is why this prayer is so important for these days. We live in a world that has lost its sense of value. It is as if somebody is switching price tags. The things that really ought to matter and have high value have low value, and the things that are ridiculously unimportant have incredibly high price tags!

So, what do you do? Take the second step and tell God, "I want to build a foundation of love, but not just any love: I want it to be with knowledge and discernment that I build this foundation on what is excellent."

3. You may be pure and blameless for the day of Christ.

This third step comes after you take the first two steps and start living for purposes that matter. As a result of that, something starts happening to you—and Christ starts being formed in you. I love the way Paul expresses it in the Philippians letter at this point: "That our life may be pure and blameless for the day of Christ, filled with the fruit of righteousness that comes through Jesus Christ" (vv. 10-11).

The words "pure" and "blameless" are very important. The word "pure" has a sense of something under the light. When you stand before Jesus on that day—the day of Christ, you will be under the light.

Here is my theory: We all look good in the dark. I look great in the darkness. But when the light comes on, you and I may not look as great as we did before. Another example would be that a particular shirt looks great in the closet when the light is off. But when you pull it out into the light, it is wrinkled and has stuff on it. And that's the point: One day the light will come on.

The word "pure" means *"Lord, what you see is what you get."* My favorite definition of a hypocrite is somebody who is not himself on Sunday. Does that register? It means that we aren't pure. And one day when the light comes on, Jesus is going to see stuff that nobody else saw, because we were so good at playing the game and hiding who we really are.

When my friend (also named David) and I were about 16 years of age, we went to the county fair. While we were walking around the fair grounds there in Arkansas, I noticed a big old pile of hay. I looked at him and said, "Hey, let's jump in the middle of it." He said, "Okay." I said, "Let's make it a race. I am going to count to three, and the first one in the pile of hay wins." "Okay, you are on!"

One, two, three . . . and we took off running. But for some reason, at the last moment, instead of jumping in the hay, I turned and ran by it. [You need to know this before I explain what happened next. The stock barns were near by, and you know what's left after the stock is gone. They shovel it up, put it in a big pile, and take hay to cover it up to keep the odor down and flies away.] Back to the story: About the time I turned, my friend takes off flying in the air and lands up to his waist in the pile of . . . . It was fresh and nasty!

When he came up, he yelled, "You knew!" I said, "I promise you, I had no idea! But you just jumped in a pile of stuff." It was hilarious!

And I promise you that on the day of Jesus Christ, he is going to pull back the hay and reveal what's really underneath in our hearts and lives. Does that communicate?

The word "blameless" means "I didn't stumble or cause others to stumble." How do you do that? How do you live a life that doesn't cause others to stumble? How do you live a life that is pure? There is only one answer: You are "filled with the fruit of righteousness that comes through Jesus Christ" (v. 11). What a cool thing! When Jesus came into your life, he is in you. One of Paul's favorite observations is, "You are now in Christ and Christ is in you." Now that Christ is in you, his life has to be lived out through you. That is the fruit of the righteousness of Christ.

I could tell you, "Go out there and be blameless. Go out there and really try hard to be pure." All the effort in the world will not make you pure. However, the blood of Jesus Christ and the life of Christ in us are what make us pure. When God the Father looks at you, he sees the Son in our life. He sees the righteousness of Christ coming out. And it is Christ's righteousness in us that will bring "the glory and praise of God" (v. 11).

Basically, this prayer is saying, "I want to start with knowledge and discernment so that my love grows in the right direction, and so that I know what matters. Then I will be pure and blameless on that Day. I will begin to look just like Jesus, and to have the fruit of righteousness that comes from him." And it all results in "the glory and praise of God."

The end of that prayer is that your life will bring praise and glory to the one who created you, the one who formed you, and the one who gave himself for you. Wouldn't it be neat if you knew that one day—when you stand before him, he would say to you, *"Well done!"* and be glorified by your life? The choice is yours.

I
CAN!

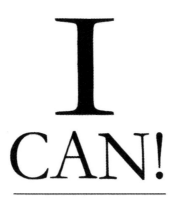

Truth #2:
I can handle all things.
Philippians 2:5-11; 4:11*b*-13

God has gone to extreme measures to help you say "I can!" and know that you really can. If you are struggling with I-can't-anymore thinking, take a close look at the scriptural passage Philippians 2:5-11:

Have this mind among yourselves, which is yours in Christ Jesus, who, though he was in the form of God, did not count equality with God a thing to be grasped, but made himself nothing, taking the form of a servant, being born in the likeness of men. And being found in human form, he humbled himself by becoming obedient to the point of death, even death on a cross. Therefore God has highly exalted him and bestowed on him the name that is above every name, so that at the name of Jesus every knee should bow, in heaven and on earth and under the earth, and every tongue confess that Jesus Christ is Lord, to the glory of God the Father.

The thing that is most important in believing *I can do all things through Christ* (Phil. 4:13) is the biblical example of what Jesus did for you. Philippians 2:6-11 describes the extent to which God would go to provide you the resources and strength you need to be successful in being able to change and do what he has asked you to do.

This Philippians passage is called *The Song of Christ*, and is simply a song the early church would sing to praise the person and work of the incarnate Christ. This Christ hymn is an outgrowth of the Old Testament praise song with its object of praise specifically being Christ. *The Song of Christ* tells the story of Jesus from the time the Son of God left his heavenly position to become a lowly, despised human and suffered a humiliating death as the sacrifice for our sin (vv. 6-8) to the time after his victory over sin and the grave when he was exalted by God the Father to the highest place (v. 9-11). This amazing song encapsulates the essence of why we, as Christians, can confidently say, "I can!"

No Lower Humiliation

If we were to imagine the worst thing that God could do or go through to show the enormity of his love for us—as well as show us that we can not only survive the toughest things in life, but overcome any adversity—what would it be? From what I know through biblical account, the humiliation of God the Son is the worst thing I [Marilyn] can begin to imagine. It was the most unlikely and ungodly experience for God to go through. And he did it for us, so that we can say, "I can."

None of us likes being humiliated. In fact, it is one of the worst experiences that we can go through—as well as one of those life experiences that often leaves a permanent scar on our heart and mind. When God was humiliated, it, too, left permanent scarring on him–nail scars. What was so humiliating?

There was no worse humiliation than the humiliation of Christ. This was not isolated to one single event. Rather, it was multi-faceted and went on non-stop a full thirty-three years. What did Christ's humiliation entail?

1. *The humiliation of Christ's incarnation.* The King of the Heaven chose to leave his throne to come to earth to be born in a stable and live as a man.
2. *The humiliation of Christ's suffering.* The Almighty God chose to take the form of a servant who endured physical suffering, intense hatred, human sin, and tremendous grief.

58

3. ***The humiliation of Christ's death.*** The Holy One chose to endure a humiliating passion, crucifixion, and death as payment for our sin.

4. ***The humiliation of Christ's burial.*** The Eternal Ruler chose to be buried in a borrowed tomb and continued under the state of death for a time as he bore all the punishment and shame due to a fallen mankind.

All of this is humiliating, to say the least—if the story ended here. And if the story ended here, there would be no Good News of Jesus Christ. And we would not be able to say, "I can do all things through Jesus Christ."

But the story did not end with Christ's humiliation. Christ suffered all of this to show us The Way. The Way of Christ means living a real life in a fallen world. The Way of Christ means suffering, humiliation, and death. But The Way of Christ also means living the Kingdom life of freedom, hope, and power. Yes, Christ suffered untold, unfathomable humiliation when he came to earth. However, he did so obediently and perfectly to the honor and glory of God the Father. He also did so victoriously!

There was—and is—no greater power on earth or in heaven than Jesus Christ. Christ's power comes through his perfect life of obedience to God. He was worthy of reward—and God exalted him above all others (Phil. 4:9-11).

No Higher Exaltation

Look again at verse 9 and note the first word of this verse: *therefore*. There is a principle in interpreting Scripture that whenever you see the word "therefore," see what it is there for. Here, as in many times in Scripture, it points back to what was said or the conditions of previous verses. There is a connection between what happened in verses 8-10 and what is going to be said in this verse. In this case, because of what Jesus did in his humiliation, "God exalted him to the highest place and gave him the name that is above every name" (v. 9).

The Father exalted Jesus, because he was obedient to God even unto death. Jesus was worthy to be exalted because he bore the scars of obedience. The result: "Therefore God exalted him" (v. 9).

The word "exalted" is used nowhere else in the New Testament. It was selected and used by Paul for emphasis. In the original Greek language it means that God super-exalted Jesus. God gave Jesus a position no other person occupies. He was lifted higher than anyone else. Also, this verb is in the aorist tense, which means it happened at a particular point in time. While I [David] do not know for sure the exact moment God super-exalted Jesus, I suspect it was when Jesus rose from the grave and walked out of that tomb: when he conquered sin and death. Jesus did not evade death; he conquered death. And in that moment, God lifted Jesus to the highest place that no other person occupies.

No Greater Name

God also gave Jesus a brand new name. He gave him "the name that is above every name" (v.9). What was that new name? I [David] don't think it was "Jesus," as that was such a common name. There were many others named Jesus. I think that the name that God gave him was the name and the title of "Lord." In the biblical mindset, a name was more than just a name. It reflected a person's character, position, title—who they were and what they did. And when it said that Jesus was given a name that was above every other name, there's only one name that it could be: It's the name—the title—"Lord."

When you go back to the Old Testament, Lord (Heb. *Yahweh*) is the name used to refer to God. The Jews would not call God by his name. Instead, they refered to God as *Yahweh*, which means "Lord–or master, ruler, the one who controls everything." This name is so significant because it is who Christ is now: He is King, Ruler, Master. He is not just called Lord, Jesus is Lord.

It was not the Church who gave him the name of Lord. It was God the Father who gave him that name. That name will never change. Jesus will always be Lord. Jesus alone holds that position above everyone else. And Jesus wears that title above every other title.

After Christ's post-resurrection appearance to the disciples, Thomas (who had not been with them when they saw Jesus) said to them, "Unless I see the nail marks in his hands and put my finger where the nails were, and put my hand into his side, I will not believe it" (John 20:25). When Thomas finally saw the nail-scarred, resurrected Christ, he said to Jesus, "My Lord and my God!" (v. 28). It's interesting that after Thomas proclaimed Jesus "Lord," this title was not used for anyone else in the rest of Scripture. Jesus alone owns the title of Lord. Why? Because the Father gave it to him. It is Christ's rightful place, his rightful position.

No Other Lord

We—along with doubting Thomas—proclaim him the Lord of our life. We call him King, Ruler, Master. We speak of God's exalting him. But what does that mean? What difference does that make? What is the extent of Christ's Lordship?

When God gave him the new name Lord, it was to declare for all eternity that:

1. Christ's Lordship is an absolute.

When you read this text (vv. 9-11), note how many times you see the word "every": "name above *every* name;" "*every* knee should bow;" "*every* tongue confess." Paul did this for emphasis. When I [David] read this text, I think, *This is not a questionable thing. This is not a contingent thing. This is something that is settled for all time.* Christ's Lordship is an absolute. Nothing we say or do will change what God has declared: Jesus is Lord. It doesn't matter what happens around us or how circumstances change: Jesus will still be Lord.

That is great news for no matter what changes or challenges come into your life, he is still Lord. What difference does that make in your life? Because Christ is always in control of all things, it doesn't matter what happens around you. His being the sovereign Lord is not contingent with things going right in your life. When you are facing life and you don't know what's out there for you, Jesus is still in control.

2. Christ's Lordship is universal.

At the name of Jesus every knee will bow . . . and then Paul gives us three locations: "in heaven and on earth and under the earth" (v. 10). When I read these words, it makes good sense that every heavenly being will bow. I can even understand that everyone on earth—even those who now mock him—will eventually bow and proclaim that Jesus is Lord. But the last location—

those under the earth—is much harder to comprehend. Paul is saying that even Satan and all the demons will bow at his name!

Those "under the earth" already know that he is Lord (Mark 1: 24; Matthew 8:29), even though they do not bow down to him or profess that he is their lord. However, they know their days are numbered. Satan and his demons who now torment us—who tear apart lives, marriages, and even churches—will one day bow their knees to Jesus Christ. I don't know about you, but I can't wait until Satan gets on his knees and confesses, "Jesus is Lord!"

3. Christ's Lordship is final.

History does not repeat itself. All of history will culminate at this point in time. History will come to a climax when all bow and confess that Jesus is Lord. This will be the final act and declaration of the world.

Does this mean that all will be saved at this point in time? Tragically, the answer is "no." Yes, it is true that those who were too rebellious to admit Christ's Lordship will confess it on that day. But it will be too late for them. Their time to surrender to the Lordship will have passed.

No Better Attitude

If we go back to verse 5 of chapter two, we will find this secret to being able to do all things: Our attitude should be the same as Jesus Christ." When you read that, do you think to yourself, "No way!" And you would be correct if you thought you were supposed to adjust your attitude to that of Christ's by your own strength and willpower. But that is what our key verse (Phil. 4:13) is all about: " I can do all things *through* Christ who strengthens me." And later in this book (ch. 8) we will discuss the importance of our not trying to pull off this kind of life change on our own—apart from Christ. But for now, let's focus on that towards which we are striving. And then we will figure out how we are supposed to attain it.

Let's break this Scripture (2:5) into two parts for our consideration:

1. Attitude, attitude, attitude!

Paul knew that our attitude is critical to our success in being able to say "I can" handle whatever comes my way and whatever God asks me to do in life. Paul was a changed man after his conversion—both inside and out. His outward circumstances and challenges took a dramatic turn (from being struck blind to being beaten—from being shipwrecked to being imprisoned), as did his inward person (from being an enemy of Christ to being a champion for Christ; from being proud and arrogant to being broken and humble). He experienced a major change in attitude: *I have learned to be content whatever the circumstances. I know what it is to be in need, and I know what it is to have plenty. I have learned the secret of being content in any and every situation, whether well fed or hungry, whether living in plenty or in want. I can do everything through him who gives me strength.*

--Philippians 4:11*b*-13

The secret of Paul's being able to do all things was his attitude: He had "learned to be content whatever the circumstances" (v. 11). Likewise, the secret to our being able to do all things is our attitude towards life. We have to have the attitude of Christ: No matter what life throws us, no matter what life gives us, no matter what life takes from us... we can handle it! The attitude of the Christian who understands the life of Christ in them is "No matter what, I can do all things, I can face all things, I can accomplish all things God has called me to accomplish, no matter the circumstances."

2. Same as Jesus Christ

The reason God the Son came to Earth and suffered humiliation was to show you the way you can handle all things and accomplish all things. And the reason God the Father exalted Jesus to the highest place was to give you the strength and power to do all that you need to do and all that he's asked you to do.

The incredible thought of the Philippians 2 passage as it relates to our being able to do all things through Christ is that when we were powerless and we could not come to where he was, he came to us. In so doing, he did for us what we never could have done for ourselves. And because of his showing us how and providing us The Way, we have been given the power and ability to change.

Because Christ did what he did, you can! You can do what you need to do. You can handle what you are facing. You can...

- *overcome any temptation or destructive habit,*
- *move beyond any past failure or current weakness,*
- *gain the desire and strength to try again,*
- *become the person you've wanted to be.*

In the end, the reason that we know that we can do all things through Christ is a promise from Scripture given to us about all of life:

What, then, shall we say in response to this? If God is for us, who can be against us? He who did not spare his own Son, but gave him up for us all—how will he not also, along with him, graciously give us all things?

– Romans 8:31-32

If God were ever going to hold anything from us, he would have held back his Son. But God spared nothing—not even his only Son—to show how much he is there for us. The living God freely gave all things that we will ever need so that we might say with certainty, "I can do all things through Christ!"

I CAN!

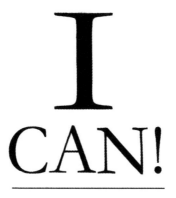

Truth #3:
I can change my thinking – and my life.
Philippians 4:8-9

I had just turned thirty and felt very dissatisfied with my life. While I [Marilyn] enjoyed the many of the trappings of a what some might have called the perfect yuppie lifestyle—plantation country club home; full social and recreational calendar; model family: devoted banker husband and adorable son; and a successful ministry career of my own—I lacked something inside me. Even though my life was so full of wonderful things and relationships, I felt very incomplete.

As I would stand in front of the congregation on Sundays leading the choral and worship music, I would feel genuinely connected to God. However, an hour afterwards—when the real-good-feel-goods of the worship experience had passed, I would begin aching inside, craving my next God-fix. I would attempt to medicate the hurt in my heart with whatever would give me instant gratification, but the need for something more just grew stronger and stronger.

Finally one day, I laid aside my pride and cried out to God in a way that I had never done before… and in a way that has forever changed my life. I was in my car driving to one of the nearby beaches to play in a morning tennis match, when I was forced to pull over my mini-van because I had begun sobbing uncontrollably. I confessed to God that although I loved him and had given my life to serve him, I had lost my passion for him. As if he did not already know what I was about to share with him, I confided that I—the church leader who inspired others to grow deeply in their faith—hated doing those things that I used to love when I was a teenager and younger adult: reading his Word, praying, spending time alone with him. I admitted that I no longer desired the things of God in the way that I craved worldly options. I had lost my heart for him. And I felt so empty and distant from God.

And do you know what this kind, gracious God did? He didn't push me away or punish me. Instead, he drew me close to him and wiped my tears with his outstretched arms. And then he did something that has forever changed my life: He changed my thinking by giving me a new desire of heart.

Up until that point in time, I had never thought to ask God to help me with the void inside of me. In my brokenness, as I reached out to him for help, my good heavenly Father put a prayer in my heart that I began to pray over and over every day for many years: *God, help me hunger and thirst for you. God, help me hunger and thirst for you.* The prayer that God placed on my heart that day changed my thinking… and my life.

That day as I lifted my head from being buried in my arms on the steering wheel, I found that I had pulled over into the parking lot of a Christian bookstore. As I got a bearing on my surroundings, it was if the Holy Spirit nudged me and said, "Go inside." I said, "Okay, God. But I don't know of anything I want to buy. If you are going to help me hunger and thirst for you, then lead me to a book that will change my life." And, within a few minutes, he did.

The book that I bought that day was by an author of whom I had never heard. However, I bought it out of obedience when God led me to it on the shelves. The book was entitled *The Holiness of God* and it was written by R.C. Sproul. I had no idea that this prayer for God to help me hunger and thirst for him would lead my family and me to leave our home in South Carolina in five years to go to seminary in Orlando where I would be a Master of Divinity student of this author, Dr. Sproul. And once at seminary, when I would be asked why I was there working on my M. Div., I would respond, "It began with a prayer that I would hunger and thirst for God, which ultimately turned into an insatiable appetite for him." God changed my thinking . . . and transformed my life.

Change the way you think.

The Apostle Paul writes that the key to life transformation is changing the way we think: *Do not conform any longer to the pattern of this world, but be transformed by the renewing of your mind* (Rom. 12:2). Our attitude and how we think directly impacts the way we live. A change in our behavior must be preceded by a change in the way we think.

We can get overwhelmed. We can begin to feel like there's no hope, no way. In so doing, we begin to focus on what's wrong and why we can't change. That's why in the Corinthian letter, Paul talks about "taking every thought captive to obey Christ" (2 Cor. 10:5). We have got to get a hold on negative, self-destructive thinking. The focus of our thoughts has to change. If you choose to believe the lies and choose to believe wrong-thinking, the only result you can have is wrong conclusions, wrong beliefs, and wrong behavior.

There is a process in our thinking that goes like this:
1. We have an event, which we will call (A), happen to us.
2. Our response to that event is what we will call (C).
3. A lot of people think there is nothing between (A) and (C), that we simply respond to a life's events or circumstances.
4. However, what they don't realize is that between (A) and (C), there is a (B), which is what we think.
5. Before anyone acts or responds to a circumstance or an event, they first think: $(A) + (B) \rightarrow (C)$
6. So the way to change (C) is to change (B).
7. You can't change (A), because stuff happens. You have to deal with life as it comes to you.
8. The way you change your response (C) to life is to change your thinking (B), because that drives what you do.

That is exactly what Paul is focusing on in Philippians 4:8-9:

Finally, brethren, whatever is true, whatever is honorable, whatever is right, whatever is pure, whatever is lovely, whatever is of good repute, if there is any excellence and if anything worthy of praise, dwell on these things. The things you have learned and received and heard and seen in me, practice these things, and the God of peace will be with you.

Paul tells us to "think on these things." And literally this is from the Old Testament idea "to meditate." After the death of Moses, as Joshua was taking leadership of the new nation of Israel, he was told by the Lord: "Do not let the Book of the Law depart from your mouth; meditate on it day and night, so that you may be careful to do everything written in it. Then you will be prosperous and successful" (Josh. 1:8).

"Meditate" is from a word that means the same as a cow chewing its cud. It means to chew on it, to think about it. To change our practices, we have to change our focus, what consumes our thoughts, how we fill our minds. We have to begin to meditate on the things that can bring us the life results we desire.

Replace poor with good.

As Christians, we are not left on our own to figure out how to do that or what to think about. In Philippians 4:8-9, we are not only told how to change our thinking, but also what to focus on in order to realize the desired change in our lives. God, through the Apostle Paul, gives us a plan that is realistic and yields impressive life results.

As we approach this passage on change, you need to understand that to change does not mean simply "to drop things from your life." (Very few of us have that kind of willpower.) Rather, you might embrace a definition of change that encompasses the idea of "replacing of one thing for another." That's how the Paul approaches change in this letter to the Philippians.

Paul encourages Christians to try a process of thought replacement. He provides the following list of guaranteed-to-work substitutions (v. 8):

- Replace lies with what is *true*.
- Switch careless thoughts for that which is *honorable*.
- Change wrong processing for *right*-thinking.
- Substitute a holy, *pure* redirection for any sinful, impure pre-occupation.
- Focus on what is of good *repute* in others rather than being hyper-critical.
- Possess a *lovely* and loving attitude rather than bitterness or resentment.

Keep practicing.

The secret to successful life-change is to change your thinking. And the secret to changing your thinking is practice. What are you to practice? In verse 9, the Paul says that you are to practice:

. . . the things that you have *learned*,

. . . the things that you have *received*,

. . . the things that you have *heard*,

. . . the things that you have *seen*.

He is speaking of those things learned, received, heard, or seen in/of the practices of Jesus Christ. These practices differ greatly from the general practices of the world, which usually are anything but pure, honorable, true, good, excellent, or praiseworthy:

But I see another law at work in the members of my body,
waging war against the law of my mind,
and bringing me into captivity
to the law of sin which is at work in my members.
–Romans 7:23

Paul goes on to explain:

The carnal mind is at enmity against God.
–Romans 8:7a

So how then can you do something that is so foreign to what you have learned, received, heard, or seen in/from the world? You begin by "taking every thought captive" (2 Cor. 10:5) and substitute that which is characteristic of Christ's way of thinking for any thing that is opposed to the mind of Christ: "Let this mind be in you which was also in Christ Jesus" (Phil. 2:5). And then you take the next thought and do the same. And then the next thought...

New habits are not learned overnight. Nor are they achieved immediately. Acquiring new behaviors requires practice, practice, and then more practice. Arthur Rubinstein, the great musician once said, *"If I omit practice one day, I notice it; if two days, my friends notice it; if three days, the public notices it."*[3] The same could be said of our Christian practices. It takes a lot of practice—persistent, consistent practice—to change the way we think and the way we act or respond.

Ask for help.

While it is up to you to practice these new ways of thinking and acting, you are not left on your own, to pull off this kind of life change by yourself. God is there to help, guide, and empower you. He promises you the very strength of Jesus Christ (v. 13) who overcame even death.

Had I [Marilyn] not broken down and shared with God those things that made my heart so heavy and my life so incomplete, I would have missed out on one of the most incredible experiences of God in my life. I couldn't keep doing life—or ministry—the way I was doing it. I needed God's help . . . and I desperately needed more of God himself in my life. My thinking changed, and so did my life.

---

[3] Source unknown.

I CAN!

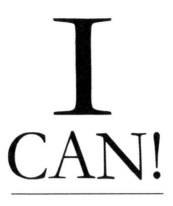

Truth #4:
I can aspire to reach heavenly goals.
Philippians 3:8-11

It may be difficult to imagine that you can become a new person or that you can live a life different from the one to which you have become accustomed. But that does not mean that these goals are unattainable. There are so many possibilities in life if you aspire to accomplish higher goals—personal and Kingdom goals.

I [Marilyn] had already lost 50 pounds when my personal trainer, George Anderson, asked me if I wanted to lose another fifty. Over the previous six months I had successfully reached my initial weight loss goal (set at 50 pounds because I thought there was no way that I could lose more than that). I had that I-can attitude working for me that day and I said, "Sure! Let's go for it!"

So I asked George, "How are we going to do it as I've begun to plateau over the last month?" He explained that we needed to shock my body by cleaning up my diet even further and by adding boxing to our workouts. Because I was encouraged by our previous success and had hope for continued success, I agreed to strictly follow his training plan—whatever would get me there.

Well, what George did not mention until a week later was a challenge for me to enter a national body makeover/body building contest. When he showed me the contest poster and presented the idea to me, I first thought, "You've got to be kidding!" But when I went home and thought it over, I loved the idea of going after a seemingly impossible goal: A 49-year-old woman, who still weighed close to 200 pounds, competing in the 35-49 age division to see who could achieve the best body results in 3 months. I came back into the gym two days later and told him that I wanted to go after this goal with the intention of winning the grand prize.

We began training twice-a-day five days a week, plus a single workout on Saturdays. My diet has never been so clean—before or since. We worked hard and smart. On the final day of the contest—when it was time for me to measure and weigh in, I had lost 5 more dress sizes (from a 16 to an 8); gone from 36.1% to 17.8% body fat; and lost an additional 41 pounds. In addition, my blood work that Dr. Samano performed on me came back with a phenomenal report. And, yes, we won the contest!

Going after and achieving that goal was transforming. It changed my life and the direction of my ministry. It helped solidify I-can thinking and goal-setting in my life. With God, anything is possible. However, we often fail to allow him to work as the trainer in our lives. We fear failure, so we don't agree to follow his training plan for our life—much less go after the big goals with which he challenges us. We don't make the sacrifices or take the risks that will help us achieve the seemingly impossible, because we forget "nothing is impossible with God" (Luke 1:37).

Philippians offers amazing insight into risking and achieving beyond-yourself goals that are only possible through Christ. In the third chapter of Philippians Paul challenges our thinking about what is truly important in this life and how we might go about attaining that to which we should aspire:
Indeed, I count everything as loss because of the surpassing worth of knowing Christ Jesus my Lord. For his sake I have suffered the loss of all things and count them as rubbish, in order that I may gain Christ and be found in him, not having a righteousness of my own that comes from the law, but that which comes through faith

in Christ, the righteousness from God that depends on faith—that I may know him and the power of his resurrection, and may share his sufferings, becoming like him in his death, that by any means possible I may attain the resurrection from the dead.

–Philippians 3:8-11

Choose the life you want.

It's up to you to choose the life you want. Of course, there are many variables. But ultimately you have to decide what is the purpose of your life. What do you want out of life? Your decisions determine your destiny. Your choices determine the shape, the course of your life—and what you become in life.

The process of choosing needs to begin with some soul-searching. Spend some time alone and apart from the distractions of your world. Ask yourself the hard questions:

- *Are the desires of my heart mostly focused on attaining possessions, power, or position?*
- *Have I lost myself in trying to be all, become all in relationships that are not as healthy as they should/could be?*
- *Do I give serious thought about—as well as serious effort to—becoming the kind of person I really want to be?*
- *What are my life goals?*
- *Where does God fit into my goals and important life choices?*
- *What does the way I live my life say about what I consider most important?*
- *Do I have a pattern of being more earthly- or heavenly-focused in my choices?*
- *What holds the greatest value to me?*

Be honest as you answer these life-defining questions. Ask God to help you see your life and your value system for what they really are: either self-centered or God-centered.

Be a new person in Christ.

When you read the book of Acts, you will see that the Apostle Paul—at that point called Saul—was forced to do this kind of personal introspection and self-evaluation. What he discovered about himself in light of God's truth (see Acts 9 and following) forever changed him. He was no longer the same. He became a new person in Christ (Paul). He was a man with a clear vision of what he could become with his eyes and heart set on heavenly goals.

Later in Scripture, in the third chapter of Philippians, Paul talks about the degree to which his life changed. He makes very clear what his new purpose in life is. He thinks back to his old self (recounting his credentials, his accomplishments, his "pedigree") and sets his new purpose in juxtaposition to the person he has become. His former life was pretty much the résumé of a Pharisee who had done very well and had been very successful. In sharp contrast, Paul makes it very clear that he has changed. He no longer lives his life governed by these kinds of choices with the purpose of elevating self. His goals are now heavenly goals: "Indeed, I count everything as loss because of the surpassing worth of knowing Christ Jesus my Lord" (v. 8). His former life is no longer what he values.

Pursue new life goals with a passion.

Paul obviously pursued his new vision, his new choices with a passion. Someone has said, "Vision does not ignite growth. Passion does. And you will never grow beyond your passion."[4] It is not enough to have a vision of where you want to go, you've got to have a passion. And that passion is best seen in Paul's language, "I consider all things but loss." This man was passionate about the new pursuits of his heart and life. Passion exudes from every verse in chapter 3 as Paul is enthusiastically stating his new-found purpose and life goal.

About what goals is Paul so passionate? In verse 8 Paul writes of laying aside his former life—all that he worked for, all that he used to consider important—for the incomparable opportunity of genuinely knowing his Lord. As we think about the words Paul uses to describe his passion, the phrase "knowing Christ Jesus" is highly unusual language for him to use to describe his relationship with the Lord. It refers not only to having a basic knowledge of his Lord, but also to possessing an in-depth, deeply personal knowledge of the Person of Jesus Christ. The language

---

[4] John Maxwell.

used here does not refer to *knowing about* Jesus. Instead, it refers to *knowing* him intimately. It's the difference between my [David's] knowing the president of the United States and my knowing my wife. I know about both of them. However, I know one only casually and I know one very intimately. Paul's first goal was to know Christ as intimately as possible.

In verse 9 Paul shares a second life goal: to have "a righteousness which comes from God on the basis of faith," not a righteousness of his own making, based on his old way of thinking (i.e., his interpretation of the Law). As a Pharisee to the highest order, Paul had lived a devoutly religious life based on rigorously following Jewish practices and laws. However, that kind of life did not lead him to a deeper relationship with his Lord or one who more and more resembled God. In his pursuit of being the best Pharisee possible, he was not growing in the righteousness of God. Instead, he was becoming more and more self-righteous.

Now, Paul passionately desires to get in a right relationship with God and to live his life based on that right relationship—not on keeping the rules and following the law as interpreted by the religious elite. He said he now pursued "not having a righteousness of my own that comes from the law, but that which comes through faith in Christ, the righteousness from God that depends on faith" (v. 9). Likewise, our goal should not just be to live a good life and keep all the rules. Instead, our chief aim should be to know Christ intimately and passionately.

Paul says to "know him and the power of his resurrection" (v. 10) is to realize that the same power that raised Jesus from the dead lives in you (Rom. 8:11). This power is a life-changing power that energizes you every day in your life and comes from that intimate relationship with Jesus that you are pursuing. He goes on to say that he desires to "share in his sufferings" and to "be made like him in his death." For you to desire likewise is just simply to realize that the former you has been crucified with Christ, and the life that you live, you live by faith in the Son of God (Gal 2:20).

Paul, the great leader, had a choice to make. He chose to be a follower. Paul chose to abandon his former glory, risk all, and passionately follow Christ. Likewise, you have a choice to make. If you choose to follow Christ passionately, you will be making the choice to accomplish all God has for you to accomplish. It's a choice to aspire to heavenly goals.

Risk radical steps to insure radical change.

As we read about how Paul pursued his new life in Christ, we see that he freely gave up all the physical, carnal, earthly things that he possessed—anything that would hinder his reaching his goals. What is shocking by today's standards is that he shows no remorse for his decisions to let go of these things: "...For whom I have suffered the loss of all things, and count them but rubbish so that I may gain Christ (v. 8*b*)." In fact, Paul compared his old life trophies to being like refuse or dung compared to his heavenly goal of knowing Christ! Compared to his choice of following Christ, everything else was secondary or without value to him. He freely gave up that which no longer was of importance to him. In fact, Paul declared that he would give up more if he had more to give.

Saul took radical measures to insure radical change. He made a choice of what he wanted in life, and refused to let anything deter him. He resolved to use "any means possible" to reach his heavenly goal (v. 11). He risked it all for Christ's sake so that he might truly know the one he followed. Saul radically changed his life and became the apostle Paul, a passionate follower of Christ.

As you examine your life in light of what you have learned about Paul, ask yourself more heart-revealing questions:

- *About what or whom are you truly passionate?*
- *What are you willing to risk in order to pursue that passion?*
- *What do you expect to be the pay-off for this pursuit?*
- *Will your reward be temporary or eternal?*
- *Are you willing to risk letting go of your life in order to passionately pursue heavenly goals?*

As incredible as the body change has been in my life, even more so has been my inner transformation [Marilyn]. As the layers of fat melted away, so did the layers of fear, doubt, hurt, anger, complacency, and self-hatred. As those changes began, I was able to replace negatives with positive steps to improve my life, my relationship with God, and my Kingdom impact. I am a new person—inside and out, because I took the risk, followed God's leading, and pursued his goals for my life.

I
CAN!

Truth #5:
I can trust God to meet all my needs.
Philippians 4:4-7, 19

It was a Tuesday morning, real early—about 6:30-ish—when the phone rang. It was one of our associate pastors, Greg, who was on vacation in the Panhandle. I answered the phone and said, "Hey, Greg, what's up?"

"David, as we were taking a walk on the beach early this morning, Sharon went into labor." He continued to explain, "David, you know it's way too early for her to deliver. We are en route to the hospital in Pensacola, and they tell us our baby is probably not going to live. And if she does live, it won't be for long. I just wanted you to pray for us."

I said, "Greg, we are going to do that, for sure. But, also, I will be there as soon as I can." I immediately left Arkansas and got on a plane to fly to Pensacola to be with Greg.[5]

I was wearing my jeans, golf shirt, and tennis shoes when I took my seat on the plane. Seated next to me was a gentleman who looked at me and asked, "You are a preacher, aren't you?"

---

[5] Happy ending to this story: Baby Rachel, who weighed only 1 pound and 15 ounces, did survive her premature entry into the world!

I don't know if we preachers have this signal that we send out that everybody picks up on, but I said, "Yes, I am."

He said, "Well, so am I. Where are you going?"

"Well, it isn't a good thing," I replied. "It is a sad thing." Then I told him the story of what this young couple was facing.

This is what he told me. And I will never forget it—even though I don't even know his name. He said, "Preacher, I have been preaching the Gospel a long time. Let me tell you what I have found. I have found there are only three kinds of people in the world, and everybody you meet will be one of those three. The first will be those who are just coming out of a storm. The second will be those in the middle of a storm. And the third will be those headed for a storm. You mark my words: Everybody you meet will be one of those three."

The longer I pastor and the longer I live, the more I find this to be true. I don't care how godly you are or how committed to Christ you are, sooner or later you will be in the middle of a storm. So how do you prepare for the storm?

Storm Preparation

Being newly transplanted to Orlando, David has just survived his first hurricane season in Florida. While this hurricane season has broken all records for producing the most tropical storms and hurricanes, it was not as bad a hurricane season as last year for the city of Orlando. My husband, Jon, and I [Marilyn] moved to Orlando from the coast of South Carolina in 1990. We had just recovered from Hurricane Hugo when we moved to the middle of the Sunshine State. We felt like we could breathe easily during hurricane season since we no longer lived on the coast.

Last year we found out how terribly flawed was our reasoning. Hurricane Charlie ripped through our downtown neighbor with winds of 100 mph. The City Beautiful lost over 10,000 trees in that devastating storm. We [Jeffcoats] lost most of our roof shingles, realized a great deal of water damage in our home, and had our yard re-landscaped when our neighbors oak tree landed over the fence and into our pool and screened porch.

We nonchalantly did some minor storm preparation for Charlie: buying the obligatory water and batteries. However, we did some serious storm preparation for the second and third hurricanes that hit us last year. We are now the owners of plywood for our windows, tarps for our roof, a generator to power our portable air conditioner, and a bunch of gas cans.

But let me tell you, as prepared as we got, by the second and especially the third hurricane, we—like so many other Floridians—were beginning to get a pretty anxious whenever we tuned into the weather channel. A hurricane party was the last thing on our mind as we were being told to hunker down for another bad storm headed our way.

So when I read how Paul tells us how to prepare for storms and all of life's needs, I listen intently. Probably you, like I, have had years in your life where the storms were not metaphorical: They were real and every bit as devastating as last season's hurricanes. And they came one on top of another. About how we should handle the storms and stuff of life, Paul writes:

Rejoice in the Lord always; again I will say, Rejoice. Let your reasonableness be known to everyone. The Lord is at hand; do not be anxious about anything.

—Philippians 4:4-6*a*

1. Don't worry; be happy.

Can you imagine what went through his readers' minds when they read the words of Paul—a man who was in prison, perhaps facing torture or execution—who told them to rejoice always… in all of life's circumstances and all of life's storms? They must have thought he was crazy to suggest such a thing!

When many of us watch the residents of the Florida Keys—who dub themselves Conchs—ride out a hurricane, we don't get it. It is as if the theme song of these long-time survivors is: "Don't worry; be happy." The same is often true when we encounter a believer who has weathered an incredibly tough life storm—a Category 5—and it's obvious that they have not been blown away. Instead, they have such abiding peace (4:7) as they rejoice in what the Lord has done to get them through the storm.

Paul writes that we, as Christians, are to live a life characterized by joy and rejoicing in the Lord: "Rejoice in the Lord always; again I will say, rejoice!" (v. 4). In this verse, Paul uses the Greek word *chairete*, which means to "be constantly rejoicing," and then qualifies this verb with the adverb "always" for emphasis. To further reiterate his point, Paul adds, "Again I will say rejoice!"

Get the point? We are to rejoice in the Lord regardless of what we are facing, for our sovereign God has everything under control—and he has a plan to get you through (Rom. 8:18-28). Our perspective of the situation at hand should be a joyful confidence in the Lord, not a preoccupation with all the bad stuff of life.

2. Don't act up; stay under control.

Paul then challenges his readers: "Let your reasonableness be known to everyone" (v. 5). The word translated as "reasonableness" is sometimes translated "forbearing spirit" or "gentleness." This word communicates the idea of your being under control—acting reasonably, not emotionally.

Have you ever been in a stressful situation—perhaps stuck in heavy traffic while running late for an important appointment—and responded more out-of-control than in-control? That's what I think this verse is all about. When life gets crazy or incredibly tough, don't act up or act out. Keep it under control—that is, under the Holy Spirit's control.

As God is in control of all things, so, too, is his Spirit living in you. When life gets stormy, let the light of God shine through you so that everyone will see God in control in you and "glorify your Father who is in heaven" (Matt. 5:16).

3. Don't be anxious; trust God.

More often than not our lives are more defined by worry and stress than by joy and peace. For many of us, an unsatisfied anxiety seems to have replaced a confident trust that God has provided the way and means to meet all of our pressing needs. Rather than responding out of faith and trust, we act out of control, full of fear and anxiety. We stress out over the uncertainty of the future and our loss of control.

In Philippians 4:6, we are told: "Be anxious for nothing." This concept is difficult (to say the least!) for most of us. Worry is what we know how to do. From childhood, we seem to have the innate ability to fixate on a situation or perceived need, and not be able to turn it loose in our attempt to get satisfaction.

Figuring out how to handle life's next crisis, the next storm, is what we struggle to do for most of our life. As we worry and fret over that which we cannot control, we become more and more anxious about how things will turn out. The Greek word *memimnao* found in verse 6 and translated as "anxious" comes from two words that literally mean "a divided mind." What Paul was saying was don't be "torn apart on the inside." And is that not what often happens? We often get torn apart by the concerns and worries of our life.

Being torn apart is not the life of joy God intends for us. Paul tells us not to be anxious about anything. We do not have to shoulder life's burdens alone. We don't have to have the solution or the "out" for every problem or storm that comes our way. Our future is not in our hands. God is in control. He is the source of our security and strength. He is the one who provides for our needs. We need to learn to trust God more than we trust in ourselves.

One of the basic ingredients of a life of joy is the ability to trust God in all things—in all circumstances for every need, in all storms for our total wellbeing. Trust is as essential to the life of the believer as blood is to the life of a body. If you bleed out, you die. If trust is lost, so is the relationship. The same is true in your relationship with God. There must be an ultimate trust that God knows your needs and will meet your needs.

Storm Survival

How do you survive the storms of life—and rejoice in the Lord while the winds are howling? The account of Jesus asleep in a boat with his disciples provides us with a survival plan:
A great windstorm arose, and the waves were breaking into the boat, so that the boat was already filling. But Jesus was in the stern, asleep on the cushion. And they woke him and said to him, "Teacher, do you not care that we are perishing?" And he awoke and rebuked the wind and said to the sea, "Peace! Be still!" And the wind ceased, and there was a great calm. He said to them,

"Why are you so afraid? Have you still no faith?" And they were filled with great fear and said to one another, "Who then is this, that even the wind and sea obey him?"

–Mark 4:37-41

How did Jesus' disciples survive the storm? They remained in the "I" of the storm. They knew and walked with the "I" of the storm. They trusted in the "I": the great I AM.

In every hurricane, there is an eye and an eye-wall. What is so amazing is that someone is crazy enough to fly into the eye during hurricane reconnaissance flights. What they tell us is that it is absolutely incredible when they get in the eye. Remember: There is still a storm, even though the conditions in the eye are calm and peaceful.

For storm survival you need to know and stay in the "I" of the storm. Jesus' disciples recognized Jesus' power over the storm when they said, "Who then is this, that even wind and sea obey him" (v. 41). If the Lord of the universe can command the wind and the sea, he certainly can take control of the forces that storm against you. And if you doubt this and prefer to worry about things over which you have no control, Jesus would ask you—as he did his disciples: "Why are you so afraid? Have you still no faith?"

It would have been great if Jesus' disciples so trusted in him and his care for them (Matt. 6:25-34), that they could have remained at peace in the storm. However, they did the next best thing: They cried out to him when they were anxious and afraid (Mark 4:38). And that is exactly what the Apostle Paul says we should do, instead of worrying:

The Lord is at hand; do not be anxious about anything, but in everything by prayer and supplication with thanksgiving let your requests be made known to God. And the peace of God, which surpasses all understanding, will guard your hearts and your minds in Christ Jesus.

–Philippians 4:5b-7

Notice what it says in verse 5: "The Lord is at hand." God is right there with you in the storm. All you have to do is stay in the "I" of the storm—and don't be anxious. And the best way to be anxious about nothing is to pray about everything.[6]

Paul uses three words for prayer: prayer, supplication (also translated "petitions"), and requests (v. 6). Why does he use three words that just about mean the same thing? Paul is emphasizing, "Let God know what is bothering you." Plead, cry, do whatever you need to do! Paul is not as concerned with the type of prayer as he is with the attitude of prayer: "with thanksgiving" (v. 6). When we give thanks, we tend to shift our focus from the problem to God. We remember that God is good and that he is bigger than any problem—or storm—that we face.

Several years ago I [David] pastored a church where there was a sweet, little, silver-haired lady named Lorraine Evans. Every time we took a group on a trip, she would show up at the church just prior to our departure. I knew this precious lady would come, step into the group as we gathered for prayer, and say, "Bro. David, allow me!" Lorraine would then recite from memory Psalm 91—and pray it as God's blessing on our journey. She well understood that we are to live in the "I" of the storm—and that I AM will watch over and care for us.

The first two verses in this psalm describe this whole idea of learning to live in the "I" of the storm: *He who dwells in the shelter of the Most High will abide in the shadow of the Almighty. I will say to the Lord, "My refuge and my fortress, my God, in Whom I trust."* The word for shelter is literally a word for "secret place." In fact, there will be some commentators who use the word "temple" as they think the psalmist is referring to the Holy of Holies in the temple. No matter how you interpret that word, what God saying is, "When you live in an intimate relationship with me, you will then abide in the shadow of the Almighty." When you dwell in the closest proximity to God, you will even abide in the Holy of Holies. Now that there is no temple structure, we are called the temple of the Holy Spirit. He now lives in us.

So, when we wake up each day, we should wake up with the awareness of his presence and say, "Thank you, Lord.

[6] Source unknown.

Thank you for loving me enough that you want me to be in an intimate relationship with you." When you live with a conscious awareness of his presence in you, you will learn the secret of living in the "I": Every day you live in the shelter, in the secret place, of the Most High God. It is a life lived in Christ, with a conscious awareness of Jesus every moment of every day of your life.

The result is that you will "abide in the shadow of the Almighty." Now this is the part that gets fun: The word for "abide," is literally the word for rest. It is also the word for endure. What does it mean to rest? It means that you are not worried; you are trusting. It means that you are totally dependent and say, "God, I know you have it under control. God, I am trusting you." Then you can rest—even as Jesus rested at the height of the storm (Mark 4:38).

That is precisely the message Paul was trying to communicate when he wrote, "And the peace of God, which surpasses all understanding, will guard your hearts and your minds in Christ Jesus" (Phil. 4:7). The result of abiding in the shadow of the Almighty—or in the "I" of the storm—is that you will have peace. Note:

1. It is the peace "of God."
"Peace of God" is used only here in the New Testament. It is not referring to a peace "with God" or a peace "from God." It is the very peace "of God." It is God himself. C.S. Lewis wrote, "He cannot give us peace apart from himself. There is no such thing."

2. It is "beyond human understanding."
It is hard for most—when they see the manifested peace of God in our lives when we are in the midst of the storm—to understand how we can be at peace. They cannot fathom how we are not worried—and, instead, we are rejoicing in what God has done.

3. It is like an army around your heart.
"Guard" is a military term. Paul is providing us with a picture of God as an army around our heart and mind. The promise of having God's peace does not mean the absence of conflict. Rather,

when the Bible talks about peace, it is presented as the Presence of God surrounding us and protecting us in the midst of conflict. God will provide for your every need.

Storm's Aftermath

If you ever wondered if God really can meet your needs, then Philippians 4:19 should be a wonderful reminder: *"And my God will supply every need of yours according to his riches in glory in Christ Jesus."* God, the Provider, will meet every need you have. Literally, this passage reads "every need of you." You can trust in God to provide for your every need.

How can God begin to make such a huge promise? This verse tells us that God will meet all of our needs "according to his riches in glory in Christ Jesus." In other words, God's ability to meet our needs directly related to his riches in glory. If there is a shortage of riches in glory, then there will be a shortage of provision for us. But we know the opposite is true: There is no shortage of his glorious riches. And to that degree, there will be no shortage of his provision for us.

Trust in the person and character of God is essential to our knowing God's provision and peace in our lives. We are promised in 1 Peter 5:7: "Cast all your anxiety on him, because he cares for you." We, as Christians, can trust God for eternity, but not for Tuesday. And how much sense does that make? Because if we can trust him for eternity, surely we can trust God for every day of the week! If we stop and think about who he is and what he has done, we should be able to put our trust in God for every need and "be anxious for nothing" (Phil. 4:6).

Oswald Chambers put it this way. He said, "The panic in your life is inversely proportionate to your faith level." In other words, the closer you walk with Him and the more you stay under the shadow of the Almighty—the more you abide in the "I" of the storm, the more peace you have.

Paul reinforces this message in another letter he wrote: *Who shall separate us from the love of Christ? Shall trouble or hardship or persecution or famine or nakedness or danger or sword? ...No, in all these things we are more than conquerors through him who loved us. For I am convinced that neither death nor life, neither angels nor demons, neither the present nor the future, nor any powers, neither height nor depth, nor anything else in all creation, will be able to separate us from the love of God that is in Christ Jesus our Lord.*

–Romans 8:35, 37-39

It is true: Nothing can separate us from the love of Christ and the love of our God, the "I" of the storm!

I CAN!

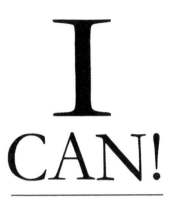

Truth #6:
I can press on to pursue the goal.
Philippians 3:12-14

Back in the days when I was pastoring in Texas and teaching at Southwestern Seminary, I [David] worked with the youth. Some students came to me one day and said, "Hey, David, there is a new ride is open at Six Flags. Can we have a youth trip? We want to go ride the Shock Wave!"

I said, "Sure!" So, my wife, Rachel, and I planned a trip and took them to Six Flags.

We showed up at Six Flags at daylight so they could be the first ones in line. When the gate opened, those guys took off running to the back of the theme park. When we got back there with the students, they were so pumped. I was looking at this thing as we were going up the stairs to the platform when I saw these two loops in it. I asked, "Does this thing go upside down?"

They all exclaimed at once: "Yes!"

To which I replied, "I think I will go down and wait on you out here. And I will pray for you!"

Then they started in on me: "Oh, man, don't wimp out! Don't be a chicken!" Well, that's all they needed to say. I wasn't going to let a student call me a chicken.

I don't know if you do this, but if I am getting on a ride for the first time, I study the faces of the guys who just came back from their ride. I look at them closely to see if their arms are in tact or if there is blood anywhere. It really boosts my confidence when I see a smile on their faces.

Well, I looked at the guys getting off the thing, and they were happy. So, I got on. This kid next to me pulled the bar down and began to strap us in. Then, the Shock Wave pulled away from the platform area and started up the incline, while an ominous clicking sound. With every click you were getting closer to the heavens: Going up, up, up!

I looked up and you could see Reunion Tower in Dallas. I thought, "If I can see Dallas, I can see Ft. Worth." I looked and I could see Ft. Worth—and the ride was still climbing. Then I looked up and there was Oklahoma City! [I am just kidding about Oklahoma City.]

When we got to the top, I panicked. I looked up and there was a catwalk at the top where they serviced this ride. I thought to myself, "How much trouble could I get in if I get off this ride. If I get on that catwalk, somebody will come get me. And the worst that could happen is that I would be thrown out of the park—and that would be a wonderful thing!" As I was thinking all of this, my seatmate kept saying, "It's okay. It's going to be all right. You can do this."

Just as the right car went over the top and took off, this kid said, "David, throw your hands up." Throw my hands up? I was afraid I would throw my breakfast up! I wasn't worried about my hands.

When we went down into that first loop, I looked over to the side and the cars were upside down on the turnpike. The rollercoaster pulled out again, went into another loop, did some more rollercoaster stuff, and pulled back into the ramp. Today, that double-looped rollercoaster is a puppy. But in those days, it was an incredible ride.

Later, as I relived the memory of this experience, I thought, "I just went on the ride of my life, but I got off the same place I got on."

Think about it… I had just gone on the ride of my life—with its thrilling drops, loops, twists, and turns—yet I got off the ride the same place I got on it. Is that not a lot like our experience of God?

Too often our going to church is like a thrill ride. The music is great, the dramas are incredible, the preacher makes you cry, and the worship makes you lift your hands. However, when it is all said and done, we walk out those doors the same way we entered. We do church like that over and over and over.

I don't know about you, but I sure don't want to keep getting off the same place I got on. I want to move ahead in my experience of and relationship with God. Likewise, it is not the desire of God that we just keep riding the ride. He wants us to make progress in our pursuit of him.

Passionately pursue God.

Paul, in his letter to the Philippians, was encouraging his readers to make progress in their pursuit of a deep relationship with God:

Not that I have already obtained this or am already perfect, but I press on to make it my own, because Christ Jesus has made me his own. Brothers, I do not consider that I have made it my own. But one thing I do: forgetting what lies behind, straining toward what lies ahead, I press on toward the goal for the prize of the upward call of God in Christ Jesus.

–Philippians 3:12-14

Note Paul used the phrase "press on" twice when he speaks of moving out in the pursuit of God. The Greek word *dioko* that is translated "press on" means to pursue something passionately. It is actually not an athletic word; it is a word from the world of sport and field. It is a hunting term. It was used in extra-biblical material to describe someone stalking or pursuing a trophy.

I am an outdoor person. My father loved to hunt. So I grew up hunting up and down the Mississippi River. One day, as a kid, I was walking through one of the hardwood bottoms along the Mississippi with its beautiful tree canopy. I looked up and the "Hartford" deer was standing there. [I am referring to the Hartford commercial with the big deer just standing there.] When the deer saw me he took off and ran away.

I followed after him. And when I got up to the trail, which was a soft, moist bottom there along the river, I could see his footprints. They were huge! So, being the hunter that I was and still try to be, I started stalking him. I was doing exactly what the word *dioko* means. I was pursuing him, following his steps right in front of me. While I couldn't see him, I knew he had been here because I could see places where his tracks had made a hole—and the water and mud were swirling around in it.

As I walked along pursuing this trophy, I began to feel like somebody or something was watching me. When I looked to my right, about 25 yards from me, was a hunter, who was asleep at the base of the tree. And he was snoring! I was standing there trying to decide what I should do: "If I wake him, he might shoot me." I carefully backed up behind a tree and cleared my throat.

Then he woke up and used words I hadn't heard yet: "Where in the blankety-blank did you come from?"

"I was just walking through here. I'm sorry, man. I didn't mean to bother you." I said, "By the way, have you seen anything this morning?"

"No," he said, "I haven't seen a thing!"

Remember, I am standing on the trail of the biggest deer I have ever seen in my life. Grinning, I said, "Oh, you haven't seen a thing? Huh?"

"Nope, I haven't seen a thing all morning."

"Hope you have a good day," I replied as I chuckled underneath my breath and kept walking.

You know why he hadn't seen anything? It is hard to see anything when you are looking at the back of your eyelids. How do you pursue something when you are asleep?

How do we pursue Christ when we are asleep and are not passionate about him? How do we go after Christ if we keep getting off the same place we got on? We don't... and never will. To which Paul says, "Dioko!" He's awakening us from our stupor state, and telling us to passionately pursue Christ, to go after him with all our heart.

Get a new attitude.

I want to invite you on the greatest ride of your life, on a journey that doesn't end until one day when you are with Jesus. However, before you get on board, you need to get real honest about where you presently are in your pursuit of God.

1. Acknowledge imperfection and get over it.

Look at verse 12 where Paul says, "I am not there yet. I am not perfect and I have not obtained this yet." In other words, Paul is saying, "I have not arrived, and I have a lot further to go. I have a lot more to know about Christ and a lot more to do for him." Remember: Paul is in prison awaiting his death. He doesn't know if he is going to live another day. (He gives us a clue earlier in the book that he believes God is going to give him more ministry; but he doesn't know for sure.) He has been serving the Lord faithfully since his conversion experience; however, he says, "I am not there yet."

I have news for you: If the Apostle Paul never reached the place where he could say, "I have learned all I need to learn and done all I need to do," then you and I will never get to that place either. As long as you are breathing, God is not through with you. As long as you are living, you are still on the journey. So, in your life and your heart you have to have the same attitude as Paul: "I am not there."

I like the little saying "If you are green, you are growing; if you are ripe, you are rotting." Do you know what that means? It means that if you ever think you are ripe and have made it in the faith and that you have learned everything there is to learn, look out, because you are rotting. If you stop running the race and stop pursuing the Lord Jesus Christ with passion, then you are dying. If you say, "But, David, I have matured and leveled out," then I would say to you, "You are really dying, because there are only two directions you can go: toward or away from him. You cannot stay in the same place."

God wants those who are like the Apostle Paul, who say, "I am not there yet. There is a lot more I want to know about him. There is a lot more I want to do for him." And God will bless those who are continually seeking to grow in the grace and knowledge of the Lord Jesus Christ. What a cool attitude!

2. Forget the past and move on.

The most important component of a successful life's journey is making the decision to press on in spite of the past or present. In verse 13, Paul writes: *This one thing I do, forgetting what is behind and straining toward what is ahead.* He said, "this one thing," and then gave us two things. Did he say this because he couldn't count? [Note: Those two things are participles in the present tense, which means you always keep doing those things.] There are three kinds of people: There are those who can count and those who can't. For example, one night after preaching a revival, I was standing at the back door. This woman walked up, looked at me, and said, "Man, how tall are you?" To which I replied, "Well, Ma'am, I believe the last time I checked I was 5'-18." She looked up at me and said, "I could have sworn you were over six feet tall!"

Paul doesn't have a problem with numbers. He has it right. There is one thing we do: "Dioko." And guess what? "Dioko" is composed of two things: *forgetting what lies behind, straining toward what lies ahead.*

• **Lay aside past failures and accomplishments.** You have to put your past in the past. You may not be able to forget, but let go of it. Let go of the bad stuff. You have messed up. You may think God cannot use you again or that he is not going to draw you close to him again, because you have sinned away your days of grace. You feel like you have destroyed your spiritual walk.

Can I tell you that you are listening to the wrong voice? That is voice of the the Enemy talking to you, and not your Heavenly Father. The Enemy is trying to keep you where you are. The last thing he wants you to do is follow after Christ. He wants to convince you to stay put as you have no right ahead, because you've messed up.

Let me assure you: Jesus died to give you the wonderful privilege to run after him. Jesus died on a cross so that you could be forgiven of any and all sin you would ever commit. There is not anything you can do—or ever have done—that will make his love and grace ineffective in your life.

If you are thinking, "I am ready to passionately pursue God again. I have been sitting back in the guilt and shame of my

92

life, and I am sick of it. I am ready to move forward," then you can. I can promise you, you can! You are good to go. God is saying to you, "Come on! Even though you have messed up big time, press on! Forget the bad stuff. Forget the past."

By the way, who wrote this book? "Paul." What did his name used to be? "Saul." What did Saul used to do for a living? "He killed Christians!" Now, if you can top that, then we will talk. If you can't top that, don't tell me you can't get past something in your past that was bad. Paul got past—and so can you. Now that is one part of letting go of the past. But there is a second part: You have to let go of the good stuff, too. You have to move beyond "the good old days." Some of us are still living in the past because that is when we were really walking with God. That's when we were reading our Bible, and doing this, this, and this. And we are glad to tell everybody, I used to do this and I used to do that! Here's my question: "What are you doing today?"

Tiger Woods, in 1997, won the Masters by twelve strokes. Do you know what he did after 1997? He changed his golf swing! When asked why—after such a convincing Masters victory—he would change his golf swing, Tiger said, "I can do better."

You may have had a glorious past and you may have accomplished some wonderful things, but, by the grace of God, you can do better. Let go of those things, so God can fill your hands with something brand new—something more exciting and more challenging. There is nothing wrong with a great past. Thank God for it. Celebrate it. However, you need to get it in perspective. God is still on the throne and he wants to do something brand new in your life. It is not about maintaining the status quo, it is about pressing on and accomplishing even more for Christ. Don't live in the past. Put past failures and successes aside. Do not keep looking in life's rearview mirror. Look at what is ahead of you.

• **Keep your goal in sight.** When Paul says, "...straining toward what lies ahead, I press on toward the goal," he is using an athletic metaphor. This is the same word that you will find whenever runners get to the finish line. What is it they do when they get right to the finish line? They will stretch and literally throw themselves forward in order to break the beam first. This metaphor (vv. 13-14) means that every fiber of my being is focused on the finish!

He used a real interesting word in the Greek, *skopos*, which sounds a lot like "scope." As a scope is something you use to get a target in sight, *skopos* (translated here as "goal"), means "mark." Paul is saying get your mark or goal in sight. Get your eyes on the target, and run for the finish line. For Christians, the mark or goal is Jesus himself. Your first goal and priority in life should be to walk after Christ.

Florence Chadwick has always but a hero of mine because I knew her story well. When I was in San Diego in the Spring, I was walking through the airport with Rachel. I looked up and they had a big poster of her; and it had her story. I didn't know she was from San Diego.

On July Fourth, 1952, Florence Chadwick set out to be the first woman to swim from Catalina Island to the mainland. It should have been no problem for her as she had already been the first woman to swim the English Channel. (She actually did it from both directions!)

She went into the icy water that day and started swimming. Fifteen hours later, after they had fought sharks off, she looked up to the boat and said, "I cannot go on." They responded, "Florence, you are less than a mile from the shore. You can do it!"

"I can't go on!" she cried. So they pulled her in.

Two months later, she went back to the same beach on Catalina Island, walked into the same icy water and swam it in a world record time—even beating the men in her time.

When asked what made the difference this time, she explained, "The second time I could see the finish." (It had been foggy on the first try. And she gave up.) Sometimes in life, it gets foggy. You can't see past the end of your nose, much less, see tomorrow. It's easy to lose sight of the goal line. However, know with certainty, Jesus is there at the finish line... cheering you on! So, too is, "the prize for which God has called me heavenward in Christ Jesus."

What is that prize? For me, it will be crossing the finish line and hearing Jesus say, "Well done, David! Way to go!" Our goal should be to run the race well—to press on and passionately pursue Christ—for the purpose of pleasing and glorifying God.

I
CAN!

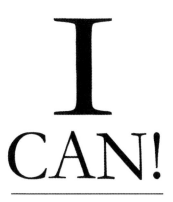

Truth #7:
I can handle anything.
Philippians 1:18-24

As I began experiencing the incredible life change that comes with losing 100-plus pounds through a healthy regime, I [Marilyn] truly felt as though I could do all things through Christ. I felt empowered! Whenever I spoke to a group or counseled individuals, God seemed to be re-directing my ministry into this area of total fitness: inside and out. Out of a growing desire to see others gain the benefits of a healthy lifestyle, Total Sculpt was born.

In the summer of 2003 I launched the first classes geared towards body and soul sculpting. The fact that I had "been there, done that" in body change gave me a lot a credibility as I encouraged these first groups of women that they, too, could do it. After each workout, we'd sit on our steppers and do that day's study. We'd talk about how God wanted to work in our lives... to sculpt us from the inside out... and our need to seek God in this process. While it was going to take a lot of discipline and hard work, we could do anything for those weeks of class in order to achieve the results we wanted. And then we would pray the most earnest prayers that God would do whatever he wanted to do in our lives to sculpt us a he saw fit.

God will sculpt your heart.

I should have watched what I prayed for—and had my friends pray for me. I should have known it was coming. If it took a year of physical training to achieve the body results that would allow me this kind of ministry opportunity, then I should have be able to reason that God was going take me through some intense soul training if I was to teach and write about how God sculpts our heart.

A couple of weeks into this inaugural Total Sculpt session, my husband and I went to the home of my son, James, and his new bride. When James opened the door to greet us, he was as pale as I have ever seen anyone. Immediately, the mom in me kicked into gear and I insisted we head to the emergency room. Three weeks and twenty-three transfusions later (as he was bleeding to death), we were given the heart-wrenching news that he had to undergo surgery that many specialists had told us was impossible. There was no way this twenty-three-year-old could survive. We faced a true dilemma: He would bleed to death without the surgery and probably with the surgery. And that reality jolt did not even take into account what all James would have to suffer and endure if he did survive.

Sitting at the surgeon's conference room table, we all felt God's control over the situation. The surgeon, Dr. Paul Williamson, was the top surgeon in his specialty—handling cases no one else would go near. While Dr. Williamson, who is a Christian, could have tried to reassure us with his outstanding track record, he, instead, told us that God is the one who had gifted him. He went on to ask, "James, are you ready to put this in God's hands?"

My son, a strong believer, accustomed to taking crazy risks for the cause of Christ—like moving to Israel when he was only 19 to immerse himself in the language and study at Hebrew University in Jerusalem—looked the doctor squarely in the eyes and confidently answered, "I am." That was it. The news we had never wanted to hear and the decision we never wanted to make had come our way, and we survived it. We weren't falling apart; in fact there was a pervasive calm that had settled over us. We prayed with Dr. Williamson, and then left . . . to await one of the toughest times a family could face.

God will answer your prayers.

What does a family say to each other in times like this? Every moment you have remaining is so precious. As my son was processing it all, he went quiet on us—which was not the way he usually related to us. That killed me as a mom as I wanted to say to my only child all those things that were important for me to say to him. And he didn't want to talk.

For you moms who may be reading this, I've got to tell you the crazy thing I did in order to cope. The day my son was to re-enter the hospital for his surgery, I insisted that he get a haircut on the way to the hospital. After three weeks of hospitalization, he was looking pretty rough. Wanting to please me, this precious kid—who was in tremendous pain—got a haircut! I know he thought that I had lost my mind. And, I guess, I probably had lost all good sense. What was my reason for insisting that he get groomed? You see, I couldn't bear the thought of his not making it through the surgery, and having someone do this to his tired, broken body after it came to rest. I just wanted to care for his needs one more time.

I experienced all of this with my first Total Sculpt group. We kept meeting and exercising, praying and bonding—especially praying and bonding—through all of this. God was sculpting my soul right in front of everyone. The body sculpting that I endured was a piece of cake compared to this kind of soul sculpting.

Here I was—teaching and being the dean at the seminary, as well as speaking and writing books on prayer—and I couldn't pray. Or, at least, I couldn't pray anything that resembled any prayers that I had prayed before. All I could do is cry out to God, and then beg others to intercede for me. I was too weak to handle this in a fine-church-lady/spiritual-leader fashion.

In my crying out to God, I would tell him how very much I hurt and how much I hated for my son to hurt. However, I did not tell God how to handle this critical situation. Even though my world seemed to be falling apart, I knew—without a doubt, without one moment of uncertainty—that God was in control of the situation. I knew that he had a plan for all of this—however he chose to handle it. The kind of faith and the degree of peace I felt could not have possibly come from me. It could have only come from God. The only thing I asked God to do was to be glorified in all of this—whatever the outcome. I begged God to work out his glory in all of our lives. While I was not emotionally ready to lose my child, I was spiritually prepared to handle anything that God chose for us to walk through.

When a physician friend came by to check on us while we were in the surgical waiting area, I asked him to go to the operating room to check on James—as it had been many hours since he went in to surgery. When Tim came out to give us a progress report, I will never forget the grave look he had on his face as he attempted not to tell us anything. And he really didn't... until it was all over.

Later Tim shared that when he went in the operating room, he encountered a frantic O.R. nurse who told him, "I wish I had never come into work today. This operating room has been a war zone." It seems they encountered one complication after another—one bleeder after another—throughout the surgery. It was touch-and-go as the surgeon and staff heroically tried to save my son's life.

God chose to be glorified that day by allowing my son to miraculously pull through. There was no other explanation—apart from God healing intervention—why James survived. And although he suffered through a year of post-surgical physical—and non-physical—torment, God held him close to his heart and restored him to incredible wholeness.

God will grant you faith that can handle anything.

I do believe God was glorified in all of this. Many have told us how God touched their hearts throughout all of this. Some could not understand the calm and the assurance that took over in our lives.

As I try to explain my perspective of this, I can think of no better scriptural passage that articulates this than the first chapter of Philippians:

What then? Only that in every way, whether in pretense or in truth, Christ is proclaimed; and in this I rejoice. Yes, and I will rejoice, for I know that this will turn out for my deliverance through your prayers and the provision of the Spirit of Jesus

Christ, according to my earnest expectation and hope, that I will not be put to shame in anything, but that with all boldness, Christ will even now, as always, be exalted in my body, whether by life or by death. For to me, to live is Christ and to die is gain.

–Philippians 1:18-21

If you have a chance, look at the verses that immediately precede this passage (vv. 12-17). Paul talks about how God has used his imprisonment to further the cause of Christ. Paul expresses a mature understanding of God's having a purpose for everything he allows in our life... and of God's using all things for our good and to further advance his Kingdom (Rom. 8:28).

As you continue reading Philippians 1 and get to our focal passage, notice these two things: the desire of Paul and the dilemma of Paul. And note that the dilemma was created by the desire.

1. The desire of Paul—as expressed in this passage—is very obvious. He wants Christ to be exalted. He doesn't want to be ashamed because his response to circumstances or for the way he lived his life when he stands before Jesus (v. 20). Instead, he wants to face his current situation—and all of life—with sufficient courage so that Christ will be exalted (v. 20).

   Before you are able to claim that exalting Christ is your one desire above all else, one thing must happen: You have to come to the place in your life where you have died to self and your will no longer rules your life. As this happens, you get to the point where it doesn't matter to you how God works in a situation. You trust him enough so that you are able to surrender your will and desires to him. Few ever get to this place in their relationship to God. Few ever are able to pray for the Lord to do whatever he wants, through whatever circumstances so that Jesus Christ is exalted. However, the only way that Christ truly can be exalted in our life is if we relinquish control of our will. Jesus demonstrated this for us when—just before he paid the ultimate price for our sin—he prayed: "Father, if you are willing, take this cup from me; yet not my will, but yours be done" (Matt. 22:42).

This goes against everything that is "self." Here we have Jesus and Paul willingly laying aside their desires and offering up their lives so that God would be exalted. Paul describes it this way, "To live is Christ and to die is gain" (v. 21). That seems backwards to most of us. Most of us would say to die is Christ and to live is gain—but not Paul. For him, living means of only one thing: Life was the means to bring honor and glory to Jesus Christ.

2. Paul's dilemma is his being torn between two possible outcomes: living or dying. On one hand, he has the desire to depart and be with Christ. On the other hand, he has the desire to stay for fruitful labor. If you continue to read this chapter, Paul actually says it is better to depart, but more necessary to stay:

If I am to live in the flesh, that means fruitful labor for me. Yet which I shall choose I cannot tell. I am hard pressed between the two. My desire is to depart and be with Christ, for that is far better. But to remain in the flesh is more necessary on your account.

–Philippians 1:22-24

The Greek word used for dilemma or "hard pressed between the two" (v. 23) is a word used in Luke for a city that has been encircled by the enemy. The city is literally under siege. The other use of the word is to describe someone being torn apart, someone who is being pulled this way and that.

Paul's dilemma came as a result of his desire. Because his desire was to exalt Jesus Christ, the dilemma was created when he weighed the possible outcomes of his imprisonment—life or death—and their potential for bringing glory to God. In Paul's mind it was settled: The cause of Christ superceded the cause of Paul. All decisions were filtered through that belief system.

Don't read me wrong: I do not pretend to possess the faith of Paul. However, I don't have to have his apostolic-level of faith in order to have a faith that is real—one that colors the decisions I make and one that allows me to handle anything. Remember the words of Christ: "I can promise you this. If you had faith no larger than a mustard seed, you could tell this mountain to move from here to there. And it would. Everything would be possible for you" (Matthew 17:20). My handling an impossible dilemma—whether I should beg God for my son to live or for God to be glorified in the way God chose—was possible because of mustard-seed-size faith (definitely not Paul-sized faith!). Because of my decision to trust God in all things, God has been changing my heart's desire over the years. And God did not abandon me in my time of need when I couldn't handle it under my own strength. He came through—and did not leave me to be ashamed . . . or without hope.

God will give you hope that will see you through.
Even with an uncertain future Paul has hope because his life is in Christ. He can't lose—either in life or death. Life on earth meant more ministry opportunities for Christ. While death meant to be present with Jesus. So Paul views his situation as win-win. That kind of faith and perspective makes Paul stand out among his contemporaries. He has an amazing ability to meet life with the attitude: "No matter what happens, I win. Because my hope and confidence is in Christ, I can handle anything."

Paul is committed to doing things God's way—and leaving the outcome in God's hands. Whether Paul lived or died, he knew that his life was in Christ—and his hope was in Christ. Of this Paul writes, "According to my earnest expectation and hope..." (Phil. 1:20). The word translated here as "expectation" means "watching with outstretched head." Paul is putting his neck on the line because he expects God to come through. And he is eagerly looking to see what God is going to do. All of his hope is in Christ, not in himself.

That is the hope that will carry us through in the uncertainty of the present. That is the hope for our future. And it is the greatest hope of all: Our life is Christ—and one day we will share in his glory.

I
CAN!

Truth #8:
I can become a new person–inside out.
Philippians 2:12-13

While on a student trip, we were riding in a big school bus with the church's name on the side. We were all having a great time when, all of a sudden, Bud Parker—the student minister whom I [David] loved—pulled the bus over to the side of the road. Then he told us teenagers to get off the bus.

When we all got off the bus and were standing on the side of the road, he pointed up to the top of the hill. Bud then informed us: "At the top of the hill is a gas station. I am going to have to ask you guys to push this bus." We all looked at each other in amazement. We were to push this huge bus to the top of the hill?

Have you pushed a school bus lately? Ever pushed one up a hill? We were all in the back pushing while Bud steered the bus. The whole time we were pushing, he was sitting in the driver's seat laughing. And we could hear him!

We pushed and pushed and finally got the bus to the top of the hill. When we got to the top of the hill, Bud put on the brakes and yelled, "That's enough! That's enough!" He then proceeded to start the bus and drive it to the gas pump. And there we were: idiots left on the side of the road. He got us good!

I have never forgotten that story—and not just because somebody "got me." That story makes me think about my life and how I have spent a lot more time pushing a school bus than riding in one. And I bet you know exactly what I mean. We spend a lot more time "pushing the bus," when God called us to get on the bus. It is a work that is already done. It is a life he has already given us. And all we have to do is get in the bus and go. Yet we continue to push the bus under our own power.

Work out your salvation.

There is only one way in which you and I can ever become a new person in Christ and manifest any of God's character in our lives—and that is through the miraculous power of the Holy Spirit who made us new creatures in Christ Jesus at the point of our salvation and who indwells us to work in and through us. Apart from the Holy Spirit's empowering us, we can do nothing: *"I am the vine, you are the branches; he who abides in Me, and I in him, he bears much fruit; for apart from Me you can do nothing"* (John 15:5). We simply cannot push this bus by ourselves.

We can change. The horrible failures of our past are behind us. As Christians, we can live in freedom because our past has been forgiven. Our present, with our continuous battle with sin, can be filled with hope because Christ paved the way for change when he became human. God has provided the way for genuine change: *No temptation has overtaken you but such as is common to man; and God is faithful, who will not allow you to be tempted beyond what you are able, but with the temptation will provide the way of escape also, that you may be able to endure it* (1 Cor. 10:13). There is an escape, a way to leave the "old us" behind.

To become the person we want to be we must cooperate with God's Holy Spirit in a life-changing process. God's life plan for us includes our living our lives in a way that is consistent with his character and our calling (and that is to glorify him in and through our lives): *Therefore, my beloved, as you have always obeyed, so now, not only in my presence but much more so in my absence, work out your own salvation with fear and trembling, for it is God who works in you both to will and to work for His good pleasure.* (Phil. 2:12-15)

One of the struggles is trying to live the Christian life on our own terms, on our own abilities. But as a believer in Jesus Christ, you have a new life in you. Paul writes that you are to "work out your own salvation." Note: He does not say to work for your salvation. The verb Paul uses here means "work out," not "work for." The difference is huge. There are a lot of people working for their salvation. Just ask the average person on the street, "What does it take to go to heaven?" They will give you a "works" answer: "You will go to heaven if you live a good life, keep the Ten Commandments, do really nice things for other people, and live by the Golden Rule."

Work for your own salvation is the "push your own bus" way of thinking. However, you cannot work enough to earn heaven. You can't do enough. In fact, it has already been done—and that is the wonderful truth of Christianity. God's Word says that it's not about your works or your righteousness. It's not about how far you can push your bus. It is about the finished work of the Cross.

Think about this: If we could work our way to heaven, then why the Cross? If you can actually contribute to your salvation by working hard at it, then why did Jesus die? If you have any ounce of works thinking in you, you have just spit in the face of Jesus on the Cross. The reason he died on the Cross was to do for you what you never ever could do for yourself.

Not long ago, Rachel and I had the privilege of going to Frankfurt, Germany, to lead a missionary retreat. While there, I was invited by the imam, (who was the leader of the local mosque), to come to the mosque and present the claims of Christ (as he knew that I had a Ph.D. and had taught at seminary). What an amazing opportunity this was!

Once there at the mosque, I met with the imam along with some men who served in some role in the mosque, as well as a good many people who just walked in. When the imam said, "Present Christianity," I did!

"Tell me about the Muslims," I asked as we began to dialogue. After a while I asked, "How do you know when you have done enough to please Allah?" I will never forget this moment or his response. As the interpreter translated for him the imam looked at me—and although I could not understand his language, but I could read his face—and said, "We don't. We live between fear and hope."

At that moment, in my spirit I said, "Hallelujah, what a Savior." For, you see, I don't live between fear and hope. I live in a place called, "Blessed assurance, Jesus is mine. Oh, what a foretaste of glory divine!" I don't have to worry or question it. It isn't about if I have been good enough or done enough as to whether or not I know I have a home in heaven. Why? Salvation is the finished work of Christ that accomplished my salvation. Salvation is a gift. I didn't earn it or buy it. I received it. Make sure you understand that Scripture doesn't say, "Work for your salvation." It says, "Work out your salvation."

Let go and let God.

What does it mean to "work out your faith with fear and trembling"? "Work out your faith" means you have to let the work that is going on inside of you find its outward expression. In other words, let what is on the inside come out. And that something that is going on inside of you is the Spirit of the Living God living and working in you. [The day Jesus Christ came into your life, you received the Holy Spirit. The Holy Spirit is simply Jesus' presence in you.] And what Paul is saying in this verse is: "Would you, please, let Christ out! Would you let him change the outside of your life?"

The phrase, "work out," is actually one word in Greek, the verb *katergazomai*. In the Greek language—as in English—there are active verbs, passive verbs, and there is something called middle voice.

- Active is when you, the subject, are doing something.
- Passive is when you, the subject, are having something done to you.
- Middle voice is when you, the subject, are doing something, but something is being done to you.

The verb "work out" is in the middle voice to indicate that in working out your salvation, you have a part but then God has a part. Isn't that cool? What a perfect balance!

What is your part? Cooperate with God, and don't hinder his work. Jesus said, "If any man wants to be my disciple, let him take up his cross, deny himself, and follow me" (Matt. 16:24). Your part is to die to self, get out of the way, and let God's light in you shine out through you. The greatest thing you could do is to die with Christ. That is the middle voice. You have a part to play and God has a part to play. That is, when we die to ourselves, he completes his work in us.

What is God's part? God's part is to fill us with his Spirit, and to pour his life through us. He is able to do for us and in us what we could never do for ourselves. When we die to ourselves and let go of the control of our life, the work of Christ begins to flow through our life. It makes all the difference. It is the difference between riding in the bus and pushing it.

"With fear (Gr. *phobos*) and trembling (Gr. *tromos*)" is a favorite expression of Paul. He uses it in three other of his writings: 1 Corinthians 2:3; 2 Corinthians 7:15; and Ephesians 6:5. In every one of those incidences, Paul uses it to describe trusting God and not self. "Work it out with fear and trembling" means "I stand in awe and am amazed that God is working in me. It is not about me: It is God's life in me." To do it with fear and trembling is to honor this incredible truth that God himself is at work in you. The Creator of the heavens and earth is actually living in you. Doesn't that just excite you? Isn't that the coolest thing?

When I think about having this kind of attitude, my mind immediately goes to a conversation that I had with seventy-year-old Mr. Webb, who had known Christ since he was little. Crying, he approached me. Thinking something had happened, I said, "Are you all right, Mr. Webb?"

"David," he replied, "I have been a Christian since I was a little boy. When will I quit crying when I think about it?" Touched by his amazement and deep appreciation of God's work in him, I—fighting back my own tears—looked at him and said, "Mr. Webb, I hope never."

Don't lose the wonder of your salvation. Keep alive the sense of awe that the God of the Universe has taken up residence in your life. He could have lived anywhere, but he chose to live in you. Does that do anything for you? That is fear and trembling!

Work it out with awe, work it out with wonder, and work it out with amazement that God is in you.

Desire and energy are God's gifts.

Let's take "working out your salvation" to the next step where Paul takes it, so that it makes sense why you need to let go and let God: "For it is God at work in you, both to will and to do his good pleasure" (v. 13). God is at work in you to do two things:

1. God is at work in you to give you the desire or the "will" to do his will. This means the closer you walk with him—and the more you die to self—the more your "want-to" will change. How do you know God's will for your life? It's more simple than you may think. Ask yourself, "What do you desire most to do?' I know you are thinking, "That's not an answer." Yes, it is. For if you know him and apply his Word to your life, he will put passions and desires in you so that you will know his will for your life. Truly, the best way to know what he wants you to do is "What do you want to do?" It is God who changes your will, and it is God who has given you the desire. The converse is true, as well. The reason you dread something that you have to do for God is because that is not what you are supposed to be doing. The reason you can hardly get out of bed in the morning to go do whatever it is you have volunteered to do could be that God didn't ask you to do it. If it is God's will for you to do something, you will desire to do it.

2. It is God in us changing our want-to. It is also God in us giving us the energy to do his work. In verse 13, the little phrase "to work" (Gr. *energo*) is an infinitive. It literally means "energy." God not only gives you a desire to do what he has put you on this earth to do, he also gives you the energy to do it. Paul tells us the same Spirit who raised Jesus from the dead is dwelling in you (Rom. 8:11). Is that not phenomenal? The same power that raised Jesus from the dead now lives in you! Are you living life under your own power or under God's own power?

There was a time in my life when I thought the busier I was as a pastor, the better. You know what I was doing? I was pushing the bus—I was pushing it faster than anybody ever had in that church. I had deacons and church members coming up and applauding me because I was pushing that thing so fast.

There was a godly older woman in that community who was a member of another church. She was single and spent her day reading Scripture and praying. One day, my secretary told me she called. I asked, "What did she want?" "She wants you to come by." Talk about fear and trembling, I had no idea why she wanted to see me.

I remember driving up to her house. I walked in the front door and there she was—bent over with age—with a Bible in her hand. We greeted each other. And then she put a piece of paper in my hand. She looked me in the eye and said, "Pastor, don't read that until you get back to the office. Thank you for coming by today as I know you are busy. It was good to see you."

I turned around and walked out of the house. As soon as she shut the door, I opened the piece of paper. It read, "God never promised strength for work he did not command!"

All of a sudden, I realized why I stayed tired all the time. Was it from doing the things of God? No! It was from doing the things of myself in the name of God. I awakened to the truth: Jesus doesn't say, "Push faster. Work harder." Instead, he says: "Come to me, all you who are weary and heavy-laden, and I will give you rest. Take my yoke upon you, learn from Me, for I am gentle and humble in heart; and you will find rest for your souls. For my yoke is easy and my load is light" (Matt. 11:28-30).

Compared to pushing a bus, is that not an incredible alternative for your life? Basically, Jesus is saying, "Get inside. I am driving. Let's go for the adventure of a lifetime!" Are you ready? Are you ready to stop pushing and start living?

You can change—inside and out.

You can change! You can become the person you've always wanted to be—inside and out. Because that is how your life is created: from the inside out, you must first deal with your internal issues and spiritual needs. God has provided a results-oriented, "how-to" book that can help you realize dramatic life changes: his word, the Bible.

Start with the book of Philippians, and then continue reading . . . the rest of the New Testament, and then the Old Testament. If you read with eyes and a heart wide open, you will discover so many practical truths and real-life stories that you will not be able to get this book, his Word, out of your mind. When that happens, be sensitive and open to what God is doing inside of you. Pay close attention to what the Holy Spirit is trying to "work out" in your life as he causes you to meditate on a particular scriptural passage.

Remember: "Work out" is a verb in the middle voice, which means together you and God can accomplish a truly amazing makeover in your life. Your part is to listen to God and to put into practice the teachings from his Word. Let what God is teaching you be outwardly expressed in your life. Be the person the Holy Spirit is prompting you to be: a new creation in Christ! And if you *"seek first the Kingdom of God and his righteousness, then all these things will be given to you as well"* (Matt. 6:33). You can become a new person—inside out.

Introduction

Appendices

Hopefully you have now come to the realization that you absolutely can do all things through Christ. The key to any lasting change depends not on ourselves, but on the strength that we receive from God. However, do not use that truth as an excuse to be passive. We are called to take an active part in caring for ourselves and others. There is always more to learn about caring for God's temple.

So with that in mind, we have provided this section to assist you as you begin your journey to becoming the best you that you can be. Once you admit to yourself that you are capable of change, and are willing to put forth the effort, all that is left to do is get started. To help you do that, we have divided this section into four parts:

1. *Discussion Questions*
2. *Healthy Eating Guidelines*
3. *Journal*
4. *Authors*

Our hope is that this section will provide a little bit of tangible support. The *Discussion Questions* will help you to process everything you have read in this book, one chapter at a time. Finding a partner or a group to go through the book and questions with you would be ideal. That way you automatically have accountability, additional insight, and fellowship as you attempt to do one of the most difficult things possible: change!

The *Healthy Eating Guidelines* offer ideas for better eating. It is difficult to change our lifestyles all at once. However, small changes aren't quite so intimidating. So tackle this list one tiny change at a time. You will be pleasantly surprised at how quickly you are able to get through this list if you are seriously committed to establishing a healthier lifestyle for yourself.

The *Journal* is a great tool when starting out. You can learn a lot about your eating and exercise habits by writing them down on a daily basis. Do not approach the journal as something that will be graded at the end of a period of time. It is simply a way in which you can track your progress, and celebrate your achievements.

Finally, in the *Authors* section we just wanted you to know a little bit about ourselves. We truly believe in the biblical truth that all things are possible through Christ. Our desire is that this truth would be reflected in our lives, so that others would be continually encouraged.

Appendix A

Discussion Questions
Part One

Chapter One Questions

1. What are some things or areas in your life that you feel you cannot change? Have you ever tried to change these things before? If so, how? _____

2. Can you admit that you are where you are in your life because of the choices you have made? If possible, what choices would you un-do? _____

3. Do you believe that God has started a good work in you–and that he will complete it? How does your life reflect your belief? _____

_____

Chapter Two Questions

1. What has been your dieting experience? Have you been able to successfully stick with a healthy eating plan long-term?

_____

2. Do you really think it's possible for you to permanently change your exercise habits? Do you think it's manageable for you to change your exercise habits just for today?_____

3. Do you believe that you truly can do all things through Christ? What has been your success in doing so? Explain.

_____

_____

Chapter Three Questions

1. What cravings are most difficult for you to ignore? When do you feel these cravings most? Why do you think you crave the things you do? _____

    _____

2. What are some healthy food alternatives you can choose at the time of a craving? Where can you keep your healthy snacks so that they are accessible? _____

    _____

3. Do you believe that that you can change the way you live? What will you attempt to change first? How will you allow Christ to help you make that change? _____

    _____

Chapter Four Questions

1. What are some areas in which your needs are being neglected? What are some needs you feel are not being met because of your schedule?_____

    _____

2. What adjustments can you make in order to have more time for yourself? What are some things you can remove from your schedule to make more time for yourself?_____

    _____

3. About what do you worry or stress out in your life? Have you given these areas over to God? Can you trust God enough to meet those needs? _____

    _____

Chapter Five Questions

1. What are some social situations in your life that revolve around food? Is there a way that you can change or avoid the negative impact they have? _____

    _____

2. What are some physical goals you have been struggling to achieve? What obstacles are standing in your way? _____

3. What are some non-physical goals you can begin to strive towards in your life? What will it take for you to accomplish these goals? _____

_____

Chapter Six Questions

1. List at least one area in which you find yourself "messing up" repeatedly? What have you tried in the past to overcome this weakness? Why do you think your attempts have not worked? _____

_____

2. Do you believe you can now overcome the obstacles in your past? What will you do differently in order to succeed?

_____

_____

3. What are some issues from the past that still linger in your life? Will you push past them in order to arrive at the "glorious finish" God has waiting for you? How? _____

_____

Chapter Seven Questions

1. Do you feel as though you have reached a plateau? List at least three ways that you personally can "shock" your body back into weight loss. Which of these options are you willing to try?

_____

_____

2. Do you really believe that you—through Christ's strength—can handle any challenge? Name one challenge that you are currently facing and how you plan to overcome it. _____

_____

3. Where does your hope lie? Do you, as Paul, believe that Christ is your very reason for living? _____

_____

Chapter Eight Questions

1. What do you most want to change about yourself? Do you believe that you are capable of making that change? How can you get started?_____

_____

2. Do positive, lasting results sound too good to be true? What kind of results are you expecting from the changes you have already implemented in your life?_____

_____

3. Do you believe that you can become a new person in Christ? Who would you like to become? _____

_____

Appendix B

Healthy Eating Guidelines

Unhealthy Food Choices

Avoid:
- Refined Sugar
    - Ice cream
    - Candy
    - Cereals
- White potatoes
    - Potato chips
- White Pasta
- White Rice
- White Flour
    - Cakes
    - Cookies
    - Pastries
    - Breads
- Corn
    - Popcorn
    - Grits
- White Fat
    - Fried Foods
- Fruit juice from concentrate
- Sodas and drinks sweetened with sugar
- Honey
- Alcohol
- Corn syrup, corn starch, & corn starch solids

Reduce:
- Amount of carbs eaten in a day
- Starches (Initially you may need to avoid, not just reduce, all bread.)
- Beans (Exception: green beans)
- Diet Sodas
- Fatty dairy products (Begin phasing milk and cheese to fat-free or lean.)
- Fatty meats
- Fatty salad dressings, mayonnaise, sauces

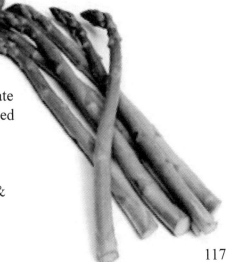

117

Healthy Food Choices

Add:

- Whole grains (Very limited)
    - Breads, cereals
    - Beware of "whole-grain" pastas
- Brown rice (Limited)
- Sweet potatoes (Limited)
- Nuts & seeds (Limited)
- Fruit
    - Berries
    - Limit bananas & raisins
- Vegetables
    - Except corn, carrots
- High-quality fats
    - Olive oil, almonds, avocado
    - Omega-3's
- Fish, fish oils
- Lean protein
    - Chicken, turkey, fish, seafood
- Yogurt (Be mindful of carb grams.)
- Water
- Fiber
- Good multi-vitamin (Use vitamins and other supplements as recommended by your physician.)

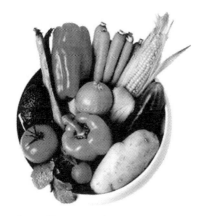

Eating Strategies for Weight Loss:

1. Eat non-veggie carbs before 3:00 p.m.
2. Quit eating 4 hours prior to bedtime.
3. Watch food combinations:
- Eat starches alone or with veggies.
- Eat proteins with veggies.
- If you eat food from the "Avoid" list, don't eat anything else 2 hours before or after eating these.

Appendix C

Journal

Spiritual Exercise Program:

30-minute-a-day plan

Choose one or more of the following spiritual disciplines to perform today as exercises to deepen your relationship with God. (Challenge: Set aside thirty minutes a day for performing these spiritual exercises.)

Retreat: Solitude, Silence, Rest
Read: Study, Meditation, Journaling
Repent: Confession, Prayer, Fasting
Restore: Guidance, Submission, Simplicity
Release: Worship, Celebration, Fellowship
Return: Loving, Serving, Forgiving

Spiritual goal(s) for today: _____
_____
_____

Prayer Journal

I am praising for _____
_____
_____

I am praying for _____
_____
_____

Physical Exercise Program:

30-minute-a-day plan

Select physical activities or exercises of your choice to perform for at least 30 minutes today. By following this plan, you will have worked out the recommended 200 minutes a week. Fitness experts have determined that for an individual to achieve maximum weight loss he or she needs 200 minutes of exercise a week.

Type of Activity: _____

Intensity: (easy) 1   2   3   4   5   6 (strenuous)

Length of Time Performed (minutes): _____

Type of Activity: _____

Intensity: (easy) 1   2   3   4   5   6 (strenuous)

Length of Time Performed (minutes): _____

Total Number of Exercise Minutes:
- Today   _____ minutes
- This Week   _____ minutes
- Weekly Goal   210 minutes

Physical goal(s) for today: _____

_____

_____

Daily Food Journal

Eating Goal: _____
_____

Breakfast: _____
_____

Mid-morning: _____
_____

Lunch: _____
_____

Afternoon: _____
_____

Dinner: _____
_____

Evening: _____
_____

Time of final snack: _____

Water:

      1   2   3   4   5   6   7   8

8–Week Body Sculpting Progress Report

Week 1   **Date:** _____

Height: _____ Weight: _____ (Circle: w/ shoes or w/o shoes)

Neck: _____ Chest: _____ Upper Arm:* _____

Waist: _____ Hips: _____ Thigh:* _____

Calf:* _____

Measure your dominant side.

Week 2   Weight: _____   Pounds Lost This Week: _____

Week 3   Weight: _____   Pounds Lost This Week: _____

Week 4   Weight: _____   Pounds Lost This Week: _____

Week 5   **Date:** _____

Height: _____ Weight: _____ (Circle: w/ shoes or w/o shoes)

Neck: _____ Chest: _____ Upper Arm:* _____

Waist: _____ Hips: _____ Thigh:* _____

Calf:* _____

Measure your dominant side.

Week 6   Weight: _____   Pounds Lost This Week: _____

Week 7   Weight: _____   Pounds Lost This Week: _____

Week 8   **Date:** _____

Height: _____ Weight: _____ (Circle: w/ shoes or w/o shoes)

Neck: _____ Chest: _____ Upper Arm:* _____

Waist: _____ Hips: _____ Thigh:* _____

Calf:* _____

Measure your dominant side.

Total Pounds Lost _____ Total Inches Lost:* _____

Make sure to multiple those items with an asterisk by two.

Appendix D

Authors

Marilyn Jeffcoat

Popular conference speaker and author, Marilyn is the former Dean of Women at Reformed Theological Seminary and former chair of the Bible Department for First Baptist/Orlando's academy. As the founder of Total Sculpt, she trains instructors, writes life-coaching curriculum, and speaks nationally. Losing over 100 pounds and transforming her life—inside & out, Marilyn has accomplished what she is now inspiring so many others to do.

Gregory P. Samano, II, D.O.

Dr. Samano is a family practice physician with a thriving practice in Winter Park, Florida. Former Chief Resident at Florida Hospital East Orlando, Samano regularly counsels people on exercise and nutrition. Having personally followed for years the eating plan he promotes, Greg has seen dramatic benefits to his own health. Active in medical missions, Dr. Samano is a Cystic Fibrosis honorary and a volunteer physician with Shepards Hope Clinics. Greg is an avid scuba diver and skier.

David Uth, Ph.D.

Highly respected for his amazing church growth success, author David Uth is co-pastor of 12,000-member First Baptist Church of Orlando, Florida. This outstanding Bible teacher (with a Ph. D. in New Testament) and former teaching fellow/adjunct faculty member at Southwestern Baptist Theological Seminary is much in demand as a national conference and revival speaker. A sports and outdoors enthusiast, Dr. Uth is a popular speaker and former board member with the Fellowship of Christian Athletes.

3 NEW Life-Changing Heart-Hitting Seminars

Total Sculpt is excited to announce Marilyn Jeffcoat's latest conference series of highly motivational seminars for your church, school, or corporate groups. These sure-to-inspire-change seminars will help participants discover their true self, re-define who they are in Christ, make extraordinary life changes, and pursue their life passion and God-created purpose. Marilyn also offers optional add-on: fun group workouts.

I Can! Workshop
Jumpstart your physical and spiritual fitness goals at the I Can! Workshop.

Come and enjoy an inspiring and provocative session with Marilyn. At the workshop, you'll learn the strategies that gave her the success of losing over 100 pounds in one year - and keeping it off!

Not only that, but you will hear about the spiritual issues that cropped up as she was losing the weight - and how she found more freedom and power in Christ than she ever thought possible. You'll be able to apply these truths to your own life to propel you to become more of who you have been created to be.

I'm Worth It! Seminar
Eight life-transforming tips to help you discover the real you and to get more out of life than you ever imagined.

Life Altaring Prayer! Seminar
You will never be the same or approach God in the same way after trying the prayer experiment and spiritual exercises this seminar teaches.

For booking information about Total Sculpt conferences, seminars, and retreats for your church, school, corporate, or leadership and staff group, contact Total Sculpt at :

1-888-9SCULPT
1-888-972-8578

Or you can inquire online at www.totalsculpt.com.